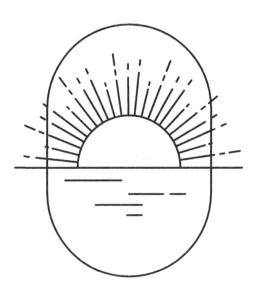

Beautiful Chaos: Embracing the Unexpected

FoundHer Series Volume Two

Soul Spark
—PUBLISHING—

Soul Spark Publishing
An imprint of Soul Spark Enterprises
soulsparkpublishing.com

This is a work of nonfiction. Nevertheless, some names, identifying details, or characteristics of individuals have been changed. Additionally, certain people who have been listed are composites of a number of individuals and their experiences.

This publication is designed to provide accurate and authoritative information in regard to the subject matter covered. It is sold with the understanding that neither the author nor the publisher is engaged in rendering legal, investment, accounting, medical, or other professional services. While the publisher and author have used their best efforts in preparing this book, they make no representations or warranties with respect to the accuracy or completeness of the contents of this book and specifically disclaim any implied warranties of merchantability or fitness for a particular purpose. No warranty may be created or extended by sales representatives or written sales materials. The advice and strategies contained herein may not be suitable for your situation. You should consult with a professional when appropriate. Neither the publisher nor the author shall be liable for any loss of profit or any other commercial damages, including but not limited to special, incidental, consequential, personal, or other damages.

FoundHer Series Volume 2, Beautiful Chaos: Embracing the Unexpected, First edition 2025
ISBN 978-1-964445-07-6 (paperback) 978-1-964445-08-3 (ebook)

Book Cover and Interior Formatting and Styling by Lucie Ward
Cover illustration by Sheviakova
Graphic icon by Marina Zlochin
Editing by Michelle Ireland

When life throws you a curve ball, gives your story a sudden plot twist,
or you have to take an expected sharp left turn...

We see you. We believe in you. We are you.

Table of Contents

Foreword		*xi*
Note to Reader		*xiii*
Sensitivity Advisory		*xv*
1.	Aging Not So Gracefully *by Carrie Scollon*	17
2.	Now What *by Tisa Sylvester*	27
3.	50/50 Chance of Suvival *by Marianne White*	39
4.	Things My Daughter Taught Me *by Marnie Law*	51
5.	The Little Alchemist MagicK *by Gwen Haas*	67
6.	A Lifetime of Shame *by Erin Gorrie*	79
7.	Inhale Love, Exhale Gratitude *by Lesa Mueller*	97
8.	Beyond the Looking Glass *by Laura Tolosi*	105
9.	Beautiful Chaos *by Miranda Pellett*	117
10.	Go Back to the Beginning *by Paula Campbell*	127
11.	Life After A Death *by Elaine De Rooy*	139
12.	Believe in Your Wildest Dreams *by Emma Lewis*	151
13.	The Hummingbird *by Heather Goodall*	165
Editor's Note		*171*
Author Listing		*173*
Acknowledgements		*175*
About FoundHer		*179*

Foreword

Dear Carrie,

I will say you threw me off this morning when you asked me to write your Foreword. After some thought, I decided I would write an "Afterward."

As I will be starting my Awesome Eighties in a few months, I've come to the conclusion that while a lot of things change, so much stays the same.

Our friendships that last over the years are one of the greatest treasures women can have. These are the girls we go through some tough and happy times with. Our paths have been so different but the results have been the same—strong and independent women. There has been love, loss, marriage, divorce, children, and dealing with mental illness. You name it and somewhere along our 70 years we have dealt with it all together.

We were the generation that couldn't Google orgasm. The birth control pill came about but a little too late for some of us! Kotex pads were wrapped in brown paper boxes hidden in the corner of the drugstore and virgins most definitely could not use tampons. Oh, and in case you're wondering, French safes (condoms) did NOT come in X-Large! After the druggist picked himself up off the floor laughing at me, it was explained they didn't come in various sizes and that was the very last favor I did my husband in that department.

Of course, we meet new friends along our way—some stay, some don't. We learn something from each one. There's always a lesson. Marriage and raising a family is not for the faint of heart. It's the hardest job we'll ever have. Mutual respect and love is something you work on every day. Yes, there's days we don't. And that's okay. I never tire of hearing Nancy Sinatra sing "These Boots Are Made for Walking" and Helen Reddy belting out "I Am Woman." I felt at the time they were singing just to me!

Back then as in now, women share the same things. Let's be there for each other.

Congratulations to our new authors for sharing their stories; sometimes a weight will be lifted and your heart will feel a little fuller in the sharing. For all our new readers, you may very well feel the same as you read through their stories.

Love you,

Mom xo (Doris McKenzie aka, Carrie's Mom)

These stories are shared with vulnerability, humility, and with great care for the readers. As some of these stories contain trauma experiences, we invite you as the reader to exercise caution and compassion and ground yourself as needed.

We have not gone into explicit detail, but some stories may be potentially stress activating. Some may make you feel uncomfortable, and once again, we encourage you to honor how you are feeling. It may mean skipping a chapter or setting it down and revisiting at another time. We have shared information at the beginning of each chapter to allow you to make the decision to continue on. Some grounding exercises if you are needing a break include placing your hand on your heart, taking a deep breath, and practicing mindfulness of where you are, what you see, what you can touch, taste, and smell. If you are activated, we trust you will seek the support you need.

Our stories are our gifts we have chosen to share, we trust you to take the wisdom and messages in each one.

SENSITIVITY ADVISORY

The following chapters may include topics that are sensitive to readers. The authors are sharing their personal experiences with trauma, grief, and terminal illness. While the details of these experiences are not explicit and are told from a perspective of healing and hindsight, please prioritize your own mental well-being when enjoying this book.

I began to let it all go, just like my waistline.

CHAPTER ONE

Aging Not So Gracefully

Written by Carrie Scollon

What in the holy hell was that!? It was hard, coarse, and prickly and it stuck out like a porcupine quill. *Was it a leftover piece of food from my breakfast, a splatter from the box of cake I just mixed up, or was it something that was life threatening?* This is what I urgently needed to know. I will never forget the day. It was such a casual motion, a whisper of my hand ever so gently on my face when I felt it. I raced through the house to my bathroom mirror and there she was... my first CHIN HAIR! I frantically searched through the million little bottles and sample sized containers, unused lipstick and brow pencils, hair ties, cotton pads, Q-tips and nail polish... okay just kidding, I rummaged through a few unopened packages of dental floss and found my beloved tweezers. I am not sure there has been a moment of such pure satisfaction as when I plucked that little sucker, never to be seen again, *or so I thought...* from my chin. This one simple little thing on my face was my first sign of what started my trip down the perimenopause lane. My hair became thinner in some areas, much thicker in others, especially on my big toes. Honestly! What in the world is the reason for that? It might just be the reason why I always wear slippers! I have now added toes to my shaving to-do list. It was small moments like this that I started to notice more and more. Aging, we all go through it but it doesn't mean we have to embrace it the same or even be happy about it. I have, from time-to-time passionately embraced this process but the minute hair started growing in places that they had no business growing in, I drew the line.

I remember *(or do I?)* walking into the grocery store thinking I didn't need a list. Really, I only needed to grab a couple of things, how hard could that be? I get up to the cashier because heaven forbid I try the self-checkout that always takes way longer when I accidentally place my bag on it and the alarms start going off. The attendant usually ends up doing it for me anyways, so I make the conscious decision, moving forward to cut out the middle man! They patiently wait as I search for the points card. I have more crap in my bag than ever before. I, of course, have the large tote because after three kids and carrying around diaper bags half my life, my brain hasn't reset to a smaller version that doesn't hold shit I don't need. I have four types of ChapStick, I have hand cream, moisturizer *(things are drying up as I write this)*, three pairs of reading glasses, hand sanitizer, fifteen... no sixteen pens, a spare tampon *(you know, just in case)*, breath mints, breath spray, a notebook, tissue, Advil, a PILL CASE *(when did that happen?!)* sunglasses, water bottle, dental floss, spare pair of undies, and last but not least my MY BELOVED TWEEZERS. Finally, I find what I am looking for, apologize to the cashier, pay my bill, and begin the search once again, for my car keys, which I find are actually in my hand.

But in seriousness, this is the reality of forgetfulness to me. All of the above happens daily and has been for many years. It scares me. How do we know when forgetfulness is a bigger issue? How do we know that it's not a genetic issue and more importantly, how do we not drive ourselves crazy wondering if this will be our future? I have a good friend who once told me that if you walk into the basement and forget why you went down there, you're doing okay. If you walk into the basement and forget how to get out of the basement, you may want to ask some follow up questions.

For me, I come from the ideal family. My parents are still together after sixty-two years of marriage and six kids and they are both physically and mentally healthy in their early eighties. With that said, I still have concerns over the brain fog versus deeper medical issues. At what point do we need to ask more questions about our health and when do we just breathe and live our life in the moment?

I leave the store with nothing that I came for. I unpack to find I already have a bottle of ketchup and a huge container of cinnamon to go beside the other huge container of cinnamon, and forgot the chicken that was for dinner. Speaking of dinner... How did that become the bane of my existence? If you want to see me lose my mind, go ahead, ask me what is for dinner!!! If I never have to hear those words spoken again I would be overjoyed.

Walking into a room, on a mission and completely forgetting why I was there. Backing out in reverse so I hopefully trigger the reason. Still cannot remember. I noticed that some groceries were left at the back door so I continued on, picking up empty containers and cups along the way, so I pop those in the dishwasher and realize I have the laundry soap in my other hand so I head to the laundry room. I swap out the loads and then it hits me! Something reeks in here! The gross smelling dishrag that was left in the sink, or is that me that smells? I had body odor before but this has hit a new level! Right... I went to the garage to get the stinky hockey gear to wash. I smile, so proud of myself. I remembered and I carried on, reminding myself of the children's book, *If You Give A Mouse A Cookie*. Oh! The groceries!!! *Where has my memory gone? Why can't I focus anymore? Is this normal? Anybody...*

I could have sworn I hung those pants to dry so they wouldn't shrink. Hmmm, guess not! Everything seemed to be shrinking, even my most precious cowboy boots. *How did I go up a shoe size? How did these pants get so tight? When did elasticized leisure wear invade my closet?* Rompers and dresses who knew they were so comfortable? Everything feels tight. It became a struggle to know what to wear. It was apparent very quickly that dressing in layers was a must. I wear a tank top under my sweater (which probably has a word like LOVE on it) topped with a vest and a scarf. My crossbody lululemon bag that never fits what I need and almost chokes me every time I panic to remove articles to reduce my hot flash. I know, I know there is a clip but I forget in the moment okay! I have finally realized that putting it inside my rather large satchel is the best way to go. My body is changing daily. What used to work is no longer an option. If the weight I have gained around my midsection could be moved to my bum area, which seems to have slipped to behind my knees and my calves, I would really appreciate that.

It is a frustrating situation as my confidence also goes up and down, or rather, shrinks and expands, with these realizations that my body has different needs now as well. I wear HOKA shoes for my aching feet. Not exactly the fashion statement I am going for but unfortunately these are things that I must do. High heels are no longer an option. Thankfully this generation of ladies has made it fashionable to wear cool, sleek runners with dresses and suits. I am forever grateful for that.

I remember a time when I was getting ready to head out to a function with my husband for work and I was frantically trying to prepare questions in my head to ask people during those awkward moments. I had to prepare because I wanted to control the conversations. I see now that this was out of my own insecurity of not feeling I was enough or that I belonged in those rooms. We start to see how we armor up when our weaknesses may be exposed. My weakness was not wanting anyone to think I was stupid. My own belief about myself that held me back, kept me small and actually safe in my mind for a very long time. I realize now that my armoring up has actually become my superpower. I turned my awkward weakness into curiosity. Curiosity about everything. Why I felt that way when certain things were said or experiences that made me step back in fear or shame. I just got more and more curious. It allowed me to learn so much about myself and others. People are very interesting and so am I. It has allowed me to give up the need for others validation, for the most part, and also to give up the need for worrying about what others think of me. Phew... that was a big one. I have learned that other people aren't actually thinking about us quite as much as we think they are. It has allowed me to get past the need to have the answers before the questions even came. I became the one asking the questions. What a relief! By giving up the need to control things that were never in my control to begin with, which honestly is most things, has also given me an immense sense of freedom. Recognizing that worrying is an emotion that does not serve me has freed me from wasting so much energy on things that are probably not ever going to happen anyway. I let it go, *just like my waistline*.

I have also let go of the fear of disappointing people. At my last couple of retreats, I made a point of sharing that we actually don't have a complaints department. We have a "How Can We Improve" department. Doesn't that just sound so much more inviting? Solutions, ideas, suggestions instead of complaints are welcome here.

My relationships and conversations have changed as well during this time of graceful aging. Realizing when we share our stories, including our struggles, the depth of some of the relationships grow and some of them start to fade away. This is very normal and it is okay. I read this acronym FOG: Fear, Obligation, Guilt. If this is how you feel in any of your relationships, it may be time to take a closer look at them. That is what I have done and continue to do. I don't make plans if it feels like an obligation and I don't want anyone making plans with me if they feel the same way. Our time is so precious. If I make plans with someone, it is absolutely because I wanted to, not because I had to. We also give others permission to step away as well. I step back and notice the friends who would be there in a heartbeat if anything bad were to happen, but what if something good happens? Are they supporting you, cheering you on? Interesting to consider that perspective as well —who shows up in the good times as well as the bad? *AKA, who can you call when the chin hair shows up, when your book hits number 1, your cute jeans no longer fit, when you are honestly so scared you're losing your mind or have had a health scare with yourself or someone you love.*

Many things are happening for a lot of us. Aging, divorces, empty nesting, loss of loved ones, aging parents. I am aging at the same speed as my parents are. Although this has always been happening, it becomes more apparent the older I get, and subsequently, the older they get. I have always felt like I am aging but my parents have stopped and I am catching up to them. Feeling like they weren't aging was a comfort for me, though I know it to be a tad bit of denial or maybe just something I didn't want to face. Being able to have candid conversations with them about the future has been extremely comforting. When we have tough, emotional conversations while we are all still in a good place, mentally and physically, it allows us to focus and appreciate our time together even more. While some things get easier and simpler, some things become a little harder through realizations that things are about to change. The only thing we ever know with certainty is that everything changes.

In a world that is filled with the need for certainty, there is only one thing we know for sure. I am going to die and so are you. With this knowledge, we have an opportunity to live this one big beautiful life as fully as we possibly can. So why is it then, that we have such a hard time doing so? Why does it feel like we only wake up when we are faced with a certain diagnosis, a loss, or a significant change? That is the question. Are we able to live this way before or without having experienced one of these setbacks? We all know eventually that we will go through something that changes our outlook on life, but why wait, why not cause a change in your outlook today and steer it rather than have it arrive on its terms? *Why is it that so many of us let life happen on autopilot versus choosing to intentionally create it?* I admittedly was on autopilot for many years and that is why I am committed to living this way of creating my life on purpose and with purpose.

Now I know that throughout my journey there were many moments where I felt unfulfilled, uncertain, and just going through the motions, but the older I get the more I can see there are periods of time that are a transition phase. One chapter to the next. From single to married, motherhood and careers to staying at home, and then like a blink of an eye, empty nesters.

That's when it can really hit home, life is happening and we are along for the ride.

I remember for myself, there were many of these moments, of course, along the way, but a big pivotal moment for me was in 2018 as I was coming on to my fiftieth birthday. Our girls were entering new phases too. High school graduations, university applications were being written and sent. Anticipation for all of us. I never really took the time to acknowledge how different things were going to be. I was still *in it*. Fully immersed in the day-to-day not looking too far ahead and what all these changes would mean for me. I was focused on all those things we ask ourselves when our children head out to enter and explore the world. *Did we do enough?* Hopefully. *Did we teach them all we could?* Maybe. *Are they ready?* Yes, more ready than we are. *Are we ready?* NO! Absolutely not. *Will they be okay?* Yes. Now I can also admit that I had moments of sadness, this phase was ending, but I also had so much excitement for what was ahead for them and for my husband and I. There was a piece of me anticipating and wondering, what's next?!

So much of my role and identity and my life had been being their mom. I also felt that along the way, beside that identity was a woman still looking for purpose. Constantly looking outside of myself for a sign, a hint of what am I here to do. I was caught like many of us are, in the busyness of life, fulfilling our roles of wife and mother, daughter, friend, sister, aunt, and all the other aspects of me, while still searching for something that was missing. A piece to the puzzle. A feeling of both, who am I now and what is next—a feeling of uncertainty and excitement all at the same time.

Maybe in this next chapter I will find my purpose to finish the puzzle of me. As I started to look at this idea of "finding" my purpose, I realized it probably began back in my twenties. Forever on the search to answer the big question: What am I here for? It took until my late forties when it hit me like a ton of bricks. What if I have been living my purpose all along? What if there was nothing to find? What if our purpose isn't something outside of us but actually all the beautiful little things and moments that we had along the way? What if it was all the car rides and carpooling conversations, the interactions with strangers, the meals? *Oh, okay, I see you side-eyeing me. I wasn't the greatest cook but still let me have my moment!* What about all the times of following the nudge to reach out to someone, offer a smile? What if it was the late night phone calls, the celebrations and connections, the being there for a friend or asking a friend for help? What if we are always *in* our purpose and that is actually enough. *What if this is it? Could I be okay with that? Can you?*

For my fiftieth birthday I knew I wanted to do something other than a big party. I wanted to create a year full of experiences. My husband named it the YOC, Year of Carrie. I loved this idea and ran with it. I made a list of fifty people that I wanted to make sure I spent time with and began the planning of something every month. It was the best year! No guilt, quality time with people I loved, and the start of honoring my time and who I spent it with. I continue to do this every year now.

Maybe this next chapter is really the chapter that I get to write and create myself. There were times I remember reminding myself that fear and excitement feel the same in our body; to take a breath and continue on even if it was scary, knowing I would be okay. I started to look at my identities, the ways I had walked through these past years, quite unaware of where it was leading me. It is a time to rediscover who we are in this new phase of life. We have grown, learned, experienced, failed, succeeded, loved and lost, and everything in between. We see the world in a whole new light when things begin to slow down.

These moments in our life, these phases, ages, these experiences—they are here to help us anchor into actually asking ourselves these big questions: Who am I now and what is next for me? By getting curious, letting go, giving up, and loving my people more, I am well on my way to feeling fulfilled and wow does it ever feel great—*this aging not-so-gracefully, or maybe I am...?*

Gotta run, Uber Eats should be here soon with dinner. *Oops did I order it?* Why are my lips so dry? Where is my ChapStick? And that better not be another chin hair I just felt.

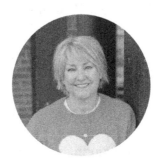

CARRIE SCOLLON

Carrie Scollon is a dynamic speaker, facilitator, and podcast host known for sparking transformation and connecting deeply and meaningfully with her global audience. Her mission-fulfilling podcast, The FoundHer Series highlights women and their stories and has been watched and downloaded around the world. Carrie consistently continues on her path of personal growth and life-long learning, sharing with her audience through retreats, workshops, summits, and group coaching. You'll find her cozied up with a cup of tea, candle, and a journal, daydreaming, creating, and always looking for opportunities to share with others that they are More Than Enough As Is. You can listen and watch The FoundHer Series podcast anywhere podcasts are heard and on YouTube as FoundHer Today.

Connect directly with Carrie at www.foundher.today.

Photo credit: LilyFire Photography

I have learned more in my life by embracing relationships and experiences that have made me feel uncomfortable than I have by sticking to the comfort of the predictable and known.

CHAPTER TWO

Now What

Written by Tisa Sylvester

At a very young age my mother left my father. We traveled on a train across Canada with a few garbage bags for suitcases. It was the three of us, my brother and I and our mother starting a new life. I watched my mom work tirelessly to provide for us. We had to utilize social security and she had to work extra jobs to keep our heads above water. I always felt loved and cared for growing up, however this was not enough to protect from the evils of society.

Four years old is when I was introduced to the justice system. I remember sitting on a cold wooden desk while an officer asked me to use the appropriate medical terms to describe sexual anatomy. When my mother found out that I was being sexually assaulted, she had no choice but to report it. Telling her had been difficult, but sitting on that desk... It became a core memory. Those are my first memories of feeling embarrassment and shame.

My youngest years were spent in a neighborhood of low socioeconomic status. I remember my friends' houses being filthy and smelling of urine and marijuana. The refrigerators were often empty. There were many stray cats and everyone smoked.

Moving forward I attended a high school where my guidance counselor suggested that high school was not for everyone. I felt so validated in that moment because I also didn't feel like I belonged in school. My best friend's mom had nicknamed me "mouse" because I would always stand in the corner of her apartment when invited in, not moving until I was told I could fully come into their space. I was in the lowest percentile for weight for my age and was very shy. I was not athletic, did not play instruments, and my report cards were a steady C average with comments of having great potential.

I dropped out of high school halfway through grade 9. I moved out of my mother's house, and I started working a job at a local pizza shop. I moved in with my much older boyfriend, paid rent, and survived on eating pizza for many years. At this time I felt successful. I was independently feeding myself, had my own space, and my own money to do what I wanted—which was mostly partying with my friends.

As the years went on I advanced to management at the pizza shop and was given more responsibility to hire/fire staff and manage other franchises while their owners were away. More responsibility came with more money. I challenged staff to upsell products and awarded them prizes at the end of the night that I bought personally. The more they sold, the more I made. I moved out of my apartment into a stand alone house, started a new relationship, got a dog, and felt like life couldn't be better. Socially and financially I felt secure and was finally very happy.

Friday nights in the shop were busy with the regular customers that would come and go. Orders always ran a bit behind schedule, but that wasn't an issue as the customers would watch me toss dough in the air for the next order and chat me up. One night as I rang up an order for a regular customer, he was complimenting my service and said, "I've seen you here for many years, what else are you working on?" I was so confused. I had to ask what he meant. He asked what I was taking in school, what my plan was from here. He asked with great conviction, "Now what?"

Until that moment I had felt really successful. I honestly thought that I had arrived in my life, like I was at the top. I was a manger, I was supplementing my own income with hard work, I was respected by my boss and colleagues, I had power in my position, and a home life that I chose with my amazing dog in a beautiful place on Vancouver Island where I could hike and swim and do whatever I wanted in my time off. I had even gotten my driver's license and a car. This was huge! The others I knew in high school were all still living with their parents. Now here's this customer suggesting I have some good potential.

Now what... That question really sat with me for some time. Driving to work one day, I had a detour which led me to drive by an old women's penitentiary. I looked up at the sign that read, "Graduate today! Come in, ask us how." I veered to the left and found myself there asking, "How?"

I felt embarrassed to now be in my twenties and admitting to anyone that the last grade I had completed was 8, but they assured me I could start in any grade I wanted. They passed me an assessment test and suggested I take it right then and there. I tried to say I'd go home and study for it and return to write it when I felt more prepared. Realistically, I likely wouldn't have returned and that would have defeated the purpose of a proper assessment to set me up for success of where I was academically right then.

One question and a left turn added advancing education to my daily routine and it felt exciting. Who knew one day I might actually graduate. Not me. I had an academic advisor who helped me pick credit courses and after about a year and a half, I graduated with honors. I felt extremely proud and so was everyone else in my social circle, including my regular Friday night customer. I loved checking in with him and his family and their positive influence.

One day my old guidance counselor from high school came in to pick up pizza and recognized me straight away. As I approached the counter he said, "Tisa!! Oh wow, how have you been? How many kids do you have now?" I was immediately insulted, only because I had just actually graduated and felt I'd done something to incorporate myself into what was considered a different class of society than I felt I belonged. I had considered having a child at fourteen with my twenty-three year old boyfriend, but my old school counselor didn't need to know that.

After receiving my diploma, I came to the office staff to thank them for making me write that assessment test the first day I came in and the dean pulled me to his office. He asked what post secondary schools he could address my letters of recommendation to and what career I had chosen. He suggested I could go into nursing as I had achieved the grades required and now had all the prerequisites. I learned that day about opportunities I had never dreamt of. He didn't say the words, but he was asking... Now what?

The dean informed me it could take as long as two years to enter into a four year program and I thought it sounded too far off to ever happen, but agreed to the letters anyway. The next day I sent them off with my applications to three universities and went back to the pizza shop. Less than two weeks later I received a phone call from a university three hours away stating they had a cancellation and if I could be ready to start in two weeks that I had a spot in Baccalaureate of Science in Nursing program.

What!? This was crazy!! Unbelievably, as informed by the dean, the bank was willing to fund this expedition into nursing with the promise to pay them back. I always thought parents had to pay for school and that this would never be an option for me. I had no idea how far forty thousand dollars would go in four years. I didn't know if it was too much or not enough, if I'd have to work through school, or live with roommates to pay bills, but I accepted the loan and carried on.

I packed up my car with a few bags and my dog and two weeks later I was on campus for a welcome BBQ making new friends. Being the "mouse" that I was, it took everything in me to walk up to a circle of people sitting in the grass eating their burgers and just sit down. Unbeknownst to me at the time, it was the circle of first year nursing students. Many of them knew each other and they started asking who I was. I made fast friends. At this moment I felt so reassured that everything would work out and that I was meant to be there.

Graduating from nursing school was a big deal. My mom, my grandparents, and my brother came for a long day of speeches, awards, and celebrations. I was one who gave a speech. It didn't hit me until I was standing in front of a theater of everyone's families, with all the faculty and my colleagues, that I probably shouldn't have sat in a pub that morning writing the speech, but, here I was again—doing something that I could have never imagined. All I could think was that I had been nominated by my classmates for the speech, so they must want to hear what I have to say. I made them laugh—in an awkward, but good way.

Four years later, now a total of six since starting my educational journey, I had received a bachelor degree. I felt sure that I had now arrived at the place we must all be destined for. Middle class. This lasted a week or so until I applied for my first job and my ego was flattened. All confidence lost as I started at the bottom of a new ladder.

I applied for my first job where I had finished my last practicum placement and was denied a position. I knew they were short staffed and hiring. This felt like a huge hit. I felt insecure and lacking confidence, and it showed. One day during my final placement, the workload was overwhelming and I couldn't find focus. I was asked to take a break by my preceptor and I went outside. I cried and cried thinking the four years was a failure and I'd never be able to do this job. I was literally hours away from finishing the program and felt like there was nothing I could do to improve at that point. I was sure my final preceptor had made the unit manager aware of my deficiencies and this was the reason I was denied employment. I felt the eyes on me as I exited that unit for the last time and felt so small.

I had to ask myself if I'd ever be ready to take on this responsibility or be able to independently manage a nursing workload. At the end of that first interview, the unit manager suggested I go north. The remote hospitals were in desperate need of nurses. She said I could come back and apply after I gained some experience. I had to respect her position as a manager of twenty years, and accept that her decisions were based on good judgment, and not personal against me. Still it felt like a popularity contest where I didn't make the cut.

In any case, I went north. Within the week my car was packed again. I was eagerly accepted as a team member with one simple phone call. I was so happy to have my first real job. I moved into a shared accommodation and worked in two remote hospitals. I worked all the hours they asked, even pulling the odd twenty-four hour shift. As for experience, unreal. The colleagues, incredible. I learned so much. I had more experience my first week than I'd have likely gained in a year or more on that structured medical/surgical unit. With no context of what the days would bring, I really had nothing to fear. I just had to show up, try my best with what I knew, and accept all the hard learning that came in stressful situations.

My life began to flourish in relationships and financially. I was so busy and after only a few weeks of work my bank account had accumulated eight thousand dollars. It felt unreal. I had never earned this much money and in such a short timeframe. I called my mom and told her. Then I bought my own bed to sleep on even had it delivered to my house. All my hard work to get to this point was paying off. I could afford to dream and I started to travel. I even took my mom on a very memorable trip to Mexico.

It didn't take long before I was chasing love and off on another adventure. Within another year or so I found myself in Alberta with the love of my life indulging in every adventure we could find. Our best adventure was having kids. My whole life I said I would never have children and here I was in my thirties having children. It was the best life choice I've made by far.

I often hear people say they are never having kids. I thought that too until I was so in love and all I could think was, I want more of you. I was also thinking that having children wouldn't change my lifestyle. That was a naive thought, but I would not change a single experience of the reality. I have lived and grown so much through having my own family. I have gained so much perspective through the experiences of my family and being part of it.

Like family, every shift in nursing brings a different perspective and experience. There is always the opportunity to learn more and do more. Many times I had found myself in critical incidents at work, doing the tasks, performing the interventions, because that is protocol for what we do. Often I didn't know why or what I could do better. I would learn more during team debriefs what could have gone better to improve patient outcomes. This was accepted as normal for a new graduate.

At this point I felt I was just part of the team doing what we should do with no insight to share. It didn't take long after graduation from nursing school until I became the senior nurse on shifts. I could only use being a new graduate as an excuse for my lack of knowledge until the next year's class graduated. The following year changed the dynamic where I was often the team leader during codes and I admittedly felt very unprepared. How was I to do patients justice by causing no harm when all I could do was listen to and follow the physician orders, without always understanding the reasoning or effects of carrying them out, or even knowing what order to do the tasks. I definitely did not feel like a contributing team member.

Years went by where I showed up and did the things on my shift and went home. In those years I was busy with nurturing a relationship and a family. After two maternity leaves and then coming to work as the senior nurse, I was feeling inadequate. Research, policies, staff—everything moved forward and I felt I wasn't keeping up. By all standards I was more than qualified, but it just didn't feel like enough. Many nights I'd stay up late researching disease processes and medications just so I could go back to work one percent better than the day before and feel more confident to answer questions and participate as a team member in patient care. I reflect on a time in nursing school when an instructor said, "You are not a nurse, a nurse is who you are." This still resonates to my core.

I wanted to BE so much more for my patients. I wanted to be present and confident. As an ongoing process, I've had to reflect on my truths and change some of my beliefs to reach any level of these two concepts—of being present and confident. It is only now in my life that when I notice a feeling like I don't belong or deserve to be in a role I've been awarded, that I start to reflect on the why behind that feeling. I always tell my students at work that no one knows what you are thinking unless you tell them. They don't know how insecure you are or that you've never done this before. I have to take my own advice. No one knows how I feel or see through me into my insecurities and history unless I tell them.

I was finding my insecurities were coming from my past. My childhood trauma, the choices I'd made earlier in my life, the lifestyle I had led, the company I'd kept, and always feeling like I didn't belong. I was feeling like there was some kind of mistake made in all the evaluations I'd been through. I was questioning if I'd somehow passed a course due to being collegial with an instructor, or if some of the open book exams were all that got me to a passing grade. I was literally feeling like an imposter. That my life had led me to where I was by complete luck and chance.

On the very first day of college an instructor asked, "Who always knew they wanted to be a nurse?" To my surprise mine was one of the few hands that didn't go up. I felt like I stumbled along this path, and then immediately felt like I wasn't supposed to be there. I judged everyone else in the room thinking they had followed the societal path of success through post secondary having had parents pay their way. I didn't think anyone there had experienced any of the things I had endured and witnessed in my life. I felt nursing school was going to be harder for *me* than it was for *them*. I definitely did not feel the class encompassed *us* as a group. I had judged others into many groups of *them* relative to what I knew about their experiences, which was actually very little.

As my classmates told stories of putting Band-Aids on dolls and how they followed family traditions with other family members in healthcare. Meanwhile, I was stuck in remembering how I learned about anatomy, and how it felt at a very young age to sit on a cold wood desk and explain it to a stranger. It felt completely random that I'd ended up in college in the first place, never mind having anything in common with my peers. In retrospect, this was me immediately distancing myself from my peers. In doing this I was not honoring others' experiences or my own. What I know now is that I have a lot to contribute coming from a unique place—as we all do. All of our backgrounds matter, and we all have something to learn from each other. Distancing myself limited what I was open to learning and limited what others could learn from me.

My life has been enriched in more ways than I can comment by being present with all different types of people and all their experiences through life and lifespan. When I started to separate the feelings of *us* and *them* and moved forward as *we*, it opened my mind to unexplored values and beliefs I had not considered before.

In college I joined a rugby team despite lacking the size and power to excel in the sport. I joined an intermediate Spanish class and immersed myself in non verbals to get by until I learned the basics. I planned and executed a trip to rural Mexico with half of my nursing class in tow. I went on remote excursions surrounded by grizzly bears. I went to a Narcotics Anonymous meeting with my Dad when he came to visit. I spent time with a Mennonite and even attended a church event. These are all experiences I would not have embraced had I continued to judge and marginalize others and myself. Some of this was very uncomfortable, but it became part of me and gave me the ability to be more relatable. I learned to ask questions. I learned what was important to other people. I am still learning.

Through all these experiences did I feel comfortable? Not at all! Very far from it. Were they all positive experiences? Ha! Also no. Some were very uncomfortable. Do I regret any of it? Also, no. When I think about regret it always comes in the experiences I missed or haven't accepted yet. I have learned more in my life by embracing relationships and experiences that have made me feel uncomfortable than I have by sticking to the comfort of the predictable and known.

Where you'll find me now is still in school. Am I still a mouse? Yes, it's a feeling that will always be there, but I feel more confident now and I know I am still developing my voice. I am aware of this feeling and ask myself why I feel uncomfortable when I get into intimidating situations. I remind myself that my past and experiences have value and that I am an important contributor to a team and within any relationship.

I took a course a few years ago where I had to direct a team of highly trained professionals in a setting where I was just learning the basics. I felt less and less sure as the case I was managing moved forward and my language became more vague with a questionable tone at the end of my statements. If I could have crawled in a hole, I would have burrowed. I was cold stress-sweating and my brain was swirling the same way as in my fourth year preceptorship when things felt so overwhelming and I was crying outside the classroom. On review of the case with the team, I was asked about how I typically present myself in these situations. The question was, "Do you command a room?" I didn't like my answer. I said yes, but only in the situations where I felt comfortable, such as with people I know, in my home, or in my usual work environment.

What a powerful question! It has resonated with me throughout my teaching relationships, but mostly in moving forward in how I use my voice and present myself. I've known I've always had to work on confidence, but never knew how or where to start. For me, starting has been approaching difficult situations and questions with honesty and doing the work to get better.

It is only now at forty-six years old that I am learning to speak with conviction. I do not have a fear of asking questions, and I never start a statement with "sorry." I say what I mean and mean what I say. I am thoughtful in what I share and strive toward. I approach problems with a solution-focused approach rather than problem-based communication. I speak more clearly now and keep an even tone.

I really hated that question, "Do you command a room?" I hated it because I had to be honest with myself, face the answer, and make a change. Change is hard. So is self reflection. But it is so necessary.

Why am I writing this now? Because I'm closer to fifty than forty and many people my age or otherwise consider themselves established, or that their window of opportunity has passed. I hear people all the time say things like it's too late to start school or learn something new. I can't just show up for a fitness class because I'm too out of shape. I don't sound educated when I speak, so I'll say nothing at all. Or simply, I could never do that. People say I could never be a nurse because they're scared of blood or couldn't tolerate seeing traumatic things. You know what?? No one *likes* that stuff. We just deal with it, and it gets easier.

Life never gets easier, it just changes and more challenges present themselves. Equip yourself with the armor you need to persevere and make the world a better place. Be confident, know your worth, and know sometimes you just have to let go of the shit that doesn't serve you. If someone doesn't value you, value yourself. If you are denied a job, know something more suitable is waiting for you. Find it. When your kid gets bullied, give or teach them the tools to know and feel their worth. When you grow your first black chin hair, electrolysis that shit before it has the chance to spread. Don't settle! And don't give up on yourself. Keep asking, "Now what," and keep going for it.

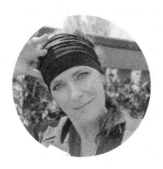

TISA SYLVESTER

Tisa Sylvester lives in Rimbey, Alberta and grew up on Vancouver Island where she continues to frequent many times per year. She is a Registered Nurse specializing in critical care. She is passionate about her work and is a dedicated preceptor. Her proudest moments are celebrated in her children's accomplishments. When she is not at work she can be found studying, or engaging in a multitude of new adventures with her family. She is a mother to two children who keep her inspired to learn and try new things. She loves the ocean and all things coastal, cooking—and even more so eating, cozy socks, travel, and time spent with friends and family. You can connect with her via Instagram www.instagram.com/tequissa.

Sometimes the bravest thing you can do is choose a different path.

CHAPTER THREE

50/50 Chance of Survival

Written by Marianne White

Imagine being told there was a fifty/fifty chance your parachute would fail if you jumped out of a plane. Most of us would hesitate, maybe even back out altogether. And yet, when it comes to marriage, we often dive in, convinced that our love story will beat the odds. But the reality is that fifty-eight percent of marriages end in divorce, and when things don't go according to plan, we're often left grappling with a deep sense of guilt and shame, as though we've failed some kind of life test. Divorce can feel like you've taken a leap without a safety net, leaving you free-falling into uncertainty.

But here's where I want to shift that perspective: what if that free-fall was exactly what you needed? What if the absence of that "safety net" opens the door to a stronger, more liberated version of yourself? Society has come a long way in talking about divorce, but let's be honest, there's still a stigma surrounding it. People often rush to judge those who choose to leave a marriage, labeling it as a failure, especially when children are involved. But divorce isn't a failure; it's a form of self-preservation and growth.

Divorce can be beautiful, necessary, and healthy. Sometimes it's the ultimate act of courage to acknowledge that a relationship, despite your best efforts, isn't serving you or your family. We live in a culture that often glorifies endurance in marriage above all else. The message seems to be, "If you just stick it out, things will get better." But sometimes, sticking it out means sacrificing your happiness, your sense of self, and your emotional well-being. It's okay to say, "Enough." Divorce can be a way to reclaim yourself, to step into a life that's more aligned with who you are becoming rather than who you were.

For me, divorce was not a defeat; it was a turning point. It wasn't about running away from problems but rather running towards a future that held more promise for myself and my children. The ending of my marriage was, in fact, the beginning of something far better—a healthier, happier version of life that I didn't know was possible until I made that choice.

I'm not advocating for divorce as a quick fix. Marriage deserves every effort and all the care you can give. You don't just "throw in the towel" when things get tough—you work through the challenges, communicate, and fight to make it work. There's incredible value in doing the hard work, especially when your marriage and family are at stake. But there's also profound wisdom in recognizing when it's time to let go. No matter how hard you try, sometimes the relationship isn't taking you where you want to go. It's okay to say, "I've done my best, but now I need to prioritize my well-being." That's not failure; that's courage.

Let's change the narrative around divorce. It's not about quitting or giving up. It's about choosing a different path—one that's filled with potential, happiness, and, often, a sense of relief. It's about allowing yourself the grace to step away from something that is no longer working for you and realizing that in doing so, you're opening the door to something better.

When it's the right choice, divorce can be the most loving thing you do for yourself and for your children. It gives you the space to heal, to grow, and to rebuild a life where you are whole again. Staying in a marriage that no longer brings joy or peace only teaches children that it's okay to settle for less than they deserve. But by choosing to leave, by showing them that happiness and self-respect are non-negotiable, you are giving them a far greater lesson.

Life isn't about rigidly sticking to a plan that's no longer serving you— it's about having the courage to change direction when needed, to seek joy, peace, and fulfillment in new chapters. Sometimes the bravest thing you can do is choose a different path. In many cases, divorce is that path, and it's time we recognized it not as the end, but as a beautiful, necessary, and healthy new beginning.

A Broken Home

"A broken home"—it's an outrageously powerful phrase, loaded with the kind of weight that can feel impossible to carry, especially during a divorce. As a society, we associate "home" with comfort, safety, and stability. Phrases like, "Home is where the heart is," "Home sweet home," or even Winnie the Pooh's gentle reminder, "Home is the comfiest place to be," conjure images of warmth and security.

But when divorce enters the picture, the term "broken home" gets thrown around, as if the act of ending a marriage shatters that sense of security and comfort. The phrase feels not only final but also inherently negative, implying something that can never be fixed. The impact is especially devastating for parents, who worry about how divorce will affect their children, fueled by a cultural narrative that paints an unfair and overly simplistic picture of what it means to come from a divorced family.

Think about the movies and television shows we've all grown up with. How often are the characters from "broken homes" portrayed as more damaged, hurt, or troubled than their peers from so-called "intact" families? It's an oversimplified narrative, one that suggests divorce leaves permanent scars on children, scars that can never heal. But it's not the whole story. Rarely do we see the other side of divorce—the resilience, the growth, the healing that can come when a toxic or unhealthy relationship ends, when people are freed from environments that weren't serving them.

This narrative becomes even more harmful when we consider what we don't hear about—the countless "intact" homes that, yes, consist of two parents, but are far from happy. Just because a family structure hasn't changed doesn't mean it's a healthy environment. Yet, these stories of dysfunction and unhappiness within married households are often overlooked. We assume that children in these homes are automatically better off simply because their parents remain together. But that's not always the case, and we rarely see it depicted in the same stark terms that we use to describe "broken homes."

When we internalize these one-sided stories from media and culture, it adds to the guilt and fear so many parents feel when deciding whether to divorce. Will my kids be hurt more because of this? Will they be labeled as coming from a broken home and face more struggles than they otherwise would? This fear is real and understandable, but it's based on a narrative that overlooks the reality that divorce can sometimes be the healthiest option for everyone involved.

I know these questions haunted me. When I was contemplating my own divorce, I was consumed by the fear of creating a "broken home" for my kids. My journal entries from that time are full of those doubts. "How can I do this to my children? Will this make their lives harder?" But what I came to realize was this: my home was already broken. That's why we divorced. We didn't have a harmonious, loving marriage. Instead, we had conflict, trauma, and emotional turbulence, none of which provided the safety or comfort a true home should.

It took time, but I came to understand that the idea of a "broken home" was a myth, at least in the way it had been presented to me. Divorce didn't shatter my home—it gave me the chance to rebuild it. My home is now filled with love, laughter, and peace. It consists of two incredible kids, two sweet dogs, a loving partner, and the happiest, most fulfilled version of myself I've ever been.

Divorce didn't ruin my life or my children's lives—it restored it. And I believe that's the narrative we need to hear more often.

Champion Divorce?

Do I champion divorce? No. I believe in marriage. I believe in love. I believe in the strength of family. I believe that relationships and marriages are hard and take work—sometimes, they require more effort than we ever imagined when we first said, "I do." But the beauty in marriage, when it works, is undeniable. A home where a wife and husband, wife and wife, or husband and husband, are selflessly in love, where they support and respect one another, and where they bring joy to each other's lives is one of the most romantic and powerful examples of love in action.

Marriage is supposed to be a partnership that lifts both people up. It's meant to be a place where each person can grow, both individually and together, through the seasons of life. When it works, it's an extraordinary bond that strengthens not only the couple but the entire family unit. It creates a model of love and partnership that children can look up to, a framework that helps them understand what a healthy relationship looks like. I will always believe in the power of a marriage like that.

But do I think we're all lucky enough to experience that kind of marriage on our first try? No, I do not. Sometimes, we enter marriages with the best of intentions, believing that love and commitment alone will be enough to sustain us. And for some, that might be true. But for many others, the reality is that love alone isn't always enough. Relationships require mutual respect, emotional safety, and shared values. Sometimes, even with the best intentions, people grow apart, circumstances change, or unhealthy dynamics begin to surface.

Staying in a marriage simply because it exists—because it's what's expected of us—doesn't guarantee happiness or fulfillment. It doesn't automatically mean you're giving your children the best possible environment. A household may have both a parents under the same roof, but if that roof is covering bitterness, resentment, or pain, is it really a home? The truth is, not every marriage can become that romantic and powerful example of love.

And that's where divorce, as difficult as it is, becomes an option that we can't ignore. Divorce is not the opposite of believing in marriage; it's the acknowledgment that not all marriages are right, healthy, or capable of providing the love and support a family deserves. It's the realization that sometimes, stepping away is the most loving thing you can do for yourself and your children.

I don't champion divorce, but I do believe in the strength it takes to make that choice when it's the right one. I believe in the courage to choose yourself and your happiness when the alternative is staying in something that's breaking you. Just because you didn't find that perfect, powerful love in your first marriage doesn't mean you won't ever find it. Sometimes, the ending of one chapter is what allows you to begin the next one, and that chapter can be filled with more love, respect, and joy than you ever thought possible.

Fighting Alone

There's a unique sadness in fighting for something you believe in, only to realize that you're the only one willing to do so. In marriage, we expect it to be a partnership where both people share the load, working through the highs and lows together. But what happens when that balance is disrupted? When one partner continues to fight, to hope, to work tirelessly to save the relationship, while the other seems indifferent, content with the way things are, or simply unwilling to try?

This situation brings a profound heartbreak. You dedicate your energy to keeping the marriage afloat, only to discover that the person you once dreamed of building a future with is either unaware of their lack of contribution or perfectly comfortable with the status quo. It's not always that they don't care; sometimes they don't recognize the impact of their complacency or find it easier to remain passive rather than engage in the challenging work of change.

For a marriage to thrive, both partners must genuinely want to work on it. No partnership is flawless all the time, but finding common ground where both parties acknowledge the need for effort and are committed to making it work is essential. When one person is fully invested while the other is passive or indifferent, the relationship is likely to struggle. It's inherently unfair to be the only one striving to mend the relationship; both partners need to share the responsibility to make progress and create a fulfilling partnership.

On the other hand, if you're contemplating divorce but haven't yet taken steps to address the issues in your marriage, be cautious of the dangerous belief that you'll simply wake up one day, back in love and eager to make it work. This mindset can create an unhealthy environment for both your spouse and your children. Constantly expressing a desire for divorce without actively working to resolve the issues only heightens uncertainty and emotional strain.

It's often through the darkest skies—through the tears, the loneliness, and the disappointment—that we begin to see the brightest stars. The end of a marriage can feel devastating, but it also opens the door to new possibilities. Recognizing that you deserve more allows you to see that sometimes, the bravest choice is to move forward and seek a future where both partners are equally invested in the journey.

A Crucial Step

I've spoken with many people, mostly women, who have gone through divorce, and it's undeniably challenging. The process—negotiations, mediations, lawyers, and dividing assets—is all messy, inconvenient, and emotionally draining. However, one of the most significant and important discussions in divorce is often about finances. In today's world, building a rewarding career and achieving financial stability are crucial, especially for women. With the reality that fifty-eight percent of marriages end in divorce, it's essential to prepare yourself financially.

Women have always been encouraged to prioritize home life and caregiving, with societal expectations and media portrayals reinforcing the ideal of women as primary nurturers. I often come across reels on Instagram that shame women for putting their children in childcare so they can work, acting like it's the equivalent of abandoning them on a deserted island. I've been there myself—many of us moms have cried in the parking lot after dropping off our kids on their first day of school or daycare. Biologically, it feels like our job is to protect and nurture them, and that mom-guilt hits hard. Even though you logically know your kids are fine, it's like there's a

44

tiny voice in your gut saying, "How could you leave them?"

But here's the thing: feeling guilty about pursuing a career shouldn't limit your options or keep you from chasing your aspirations. Supporting your kids—and yourself—is vital. So, while it's perfectly okay to feel a pang of guilt as you drive away from the daycare, remember that achieving financial stability is just as important. After all, being able to provide for yourself and your children gives you the freedom to make choices that align with your dreams, guilt-free.

Building a career and managing your finances effectively give you the freedom to make choices based on your true desires rather than being shackled by financial necessity. Imagine the power of walking away from an unhealthy or unsatisfactory relationship without worrying about how you'll pay the bills.

The Children Always Come First

My divorce, like many others, was a challenging and heart-wrenching experience. It left me navigating the uncertain waters of a modest two-bedroom condo, filled with memories of a life I once envisioned, alongside my four and two-year-old children. Those early days were a whirlwind of emotions—an unsettling mix of uncertainty and loneliness—but also a profound sense of empowerment. While my marriage wasn't meant to last, my role as a mother is a lifelong commitment that I take seriously.

In this new chapter of my life, I have dedicated myself to fostering a healthy co-parenting relationship with my ex, which is a direct reflection of my unwavering priority: the well-being of our children. I have come to understand that the traumas and wounds from my marriage are part of my personal journey. I work through them in my own time, recognizing that my healing is essential to giving my children the best possible life. This means that both Mom and Dad are present at hockey games, invited to birthdays, and actively involved in school events. Each of these moments serves as a reminder of our shared responsibility to our children, reinforcing that they are loved by both parents. This approach not only helps us navigate co-parenting challenges but also instills a sense of stability and predictability for our children, allowing them to know what to expect in their lives.

As I strive to show up for my kids in a way they can be proud of, I focus on my own well-being. I recognize that being a positive presence in their lives requires me to prioritize my mental and emotional health. When I face moments of temptation to start a fight or engage in petty disagreements—which, let's face it, can be all too easy in the heat of the moment—I remind myself of the legacy I want to leave for my children. I want them to look back on this time and feel pride in how I managed the divorce and co-parenting. I want them to see that I approached our family's challenges with grace, understanding, and an unwavering commitment to their well-being.

Ultimately, the journey of co-parenting is not just about navigating the logistics of shared parenting; it's about modeling the kind of love, respect, and resilience that I hope to instill in my children. By making their needs my top priority, I aim to create a nurturing environment where they can flourish, knowing they are cherished and supported by both parents, no matter the circumstances.

My story, like your story, is unique, and no one knows the battles you've fought. I remind myself that I don't owe anyone an explanation for my decision to get divorced. This is a deeply personal matter, and it's nobody's business but mine. I deserve to prioritize my happiness, and happiness and well-being of my children above all else. It's easy to get caught up in what others might think or say, but I need to focus on what truly matters to me. This journey is about reclaiming my life and finding peace, even if that means making tough decisions. I deserve a future where I feel valued, respected, and happy.

You matter. And your kids' well-being matters.

Divorce is not a failure, nor is it a sign of weakness. Instead, it is often the catalyst for personal growth, transformation, and ultimately, freedom. For many of us, walking away from a marriage that no longer serves us or our families is the bravest decision we can make. It is an act of self-respect and self-preservation that allows us to redefine what happiness looks like for ourselves and our children.

When I made the difficult decision to end my marriage, I feared the unknown—I feared what it would mean for my kids, for my future, and for my sense of worth. But what I learned through this journey was that divorce doesn't "break" a home; it gives you the opportunity to rebuild one. It can create a space filled with love, peace, and purpose—a sanctuary where both you and your children can thrive.

Yes, marriages are worth fighting for, but not at the cost of your self-worth, happiness, or emotional well-being. When the effort becomes one-sided, respect and shared values deteriorate, or staying feels like a sacrifice of your true self, it's okay to choose a different path. It takes incredible courage to step away from something familiar and into the uncertainty of the unknown. Yet it's within this uncertainty that you often discover your strongest, most authentic self.

This new chapter, whether you call it a "rebuilt home" or simply the next step in your journey, can be one of joy, strength, and fulfillment. Divorce, as difficult as it may be, offers an opportunity to live a life more aligned with your values, your needs, and your dreams. It teaches your children a valuable lesson, too—that it's never too late to choose yourself, prioritize happiness, and live with integrity.

As I rebuild my life, I focus on what matters most—my well-being, my boys, and the future I'm creating for us. I remind myself that I am not broken, and neither is my family. I am evolving. My love story is the one where I love myself enough to let go and move forward. Embracing this journey has ultimately led me and my boys to a life rich with joy and resilience, where hope and happiness flourish.

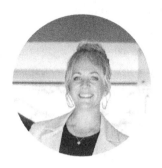

MARIANNE WHITE

Marianne Elizabeth White is an advocate for self-discovery and empowerment. Through her writing, she shares her personal journey of resilience and growth, inspiring others to embrace their worth and pursue their passions fearlessly. As the owner of an interior design firm, Marianne understands the importance of creating safe and beautiful spaces that reflect one's innermost desires and aspirations. Her commitment to helping others realize their potential shines through in her work, as she champions the power of self-love and authenticity.

Website: www.marianneelizabethdesign.com
Instagram: @marianneelizabethdesign

There is an invisible thread of connection between mother and child; and between mother and daughter a certain bond, with the shared secret of what it is to be a woman.

Sensitivity Advisory: This chapter references personal experiences of death of a child and leukemia.

CHAPTER FOUR

Things My Daughter Taught Me

Written by Marnie Law

I remember the first time I heard my daughter's heartbeat, when she was still inside of me, a small miracle in the making. There was the wonder of the thump thumping with a slight *swish* behind it, as she swam in the sea of protection my body offered. I remember the magic of pregnancy, the joy of new life held within, and the feeling that I wanted it to last forever. I remember her tiny head and the smell of her skin, how she nursed easily and snuggled generously. She was beautiful and with a reddish tinge to the blonde wisps of her downy hair, she perfectly suited her name: Christina Marie Paisley. We called her Christie.

I remember the last time I heard her heartbeat, feeling as if I was falling into an abyss as the monitors kept time, continuing to beep until the end when the merciful nurse behind the desk in the ICU turned the sound off so that we wouldn't need to hear the finality of her heart stop. I think she was already gone; I didn't see her stir. Her breath had become so slight that the rise and fall of her chest was almost undetectable. Her skin mottled as the blood left her extremities and her hands were stiff and cold. It felt as if her soul had already lifted up and away, taking those steps into the beyond where I could not follow her. The journey from the first moment to the last held a lifetime in twenty-seven years. It was not enough.

Christie was not my firstborn. My son, Nathan, was two years and three months older. When I had him, and held him in my arms, I thought I could never love another human being as much. I remember wondering what it would be like to have another child when my whole heart was wrapped up in my first. New to motherhood, I didn't realize then that love is infinite, and there is always more than enough. Our hearts expand outward with each child and other people who come into our lives. We have the capacity for so much love if we allow it.

Christie loved deeply and loved her people. She was a complicated soul, outwardly bold, and sometimes seemed a little tough, but on the inside, she was sensitive, and had a huge heart, with so much love to give. I wish I could have seen her become a mother; it was what she always wanted, to give love wholeheartedly, and to have a family of her own. I grieve my daughter, but I also mourn the loss of what will never be. She didn't have the opportunity to know what it was to bear a child. I would love to have seen her as a radiant bride with someone who adored her. I would love to have watched her experience pregnancy and birth with the joy I too, felt in pregnancy. I would love to have seen her love her baby the way I loved her.

Last year our first grandchild was born five and a half weeks early. A tiny baby so fragile and seemingly unready for the world, yet a living breathing little human with his very own personality, his spirit inhabiting his tiny body as it grew, revealing itself to the world more each day. As I see him with my daughter-in-law, I am reminded of what that bond is like between a mother and child. The closeness, the trust, the intrinsic knowing of their feelings and needs when awake and in sleep. I felt that with my own children more than thirty years ago, first with Nathan and then Christie. They reveal themselves day by day, but it is hard to prepare for them as adults, as they are forever our children. There is an invisible thread of connection between mother and child; and between mother and daughter a certain bond, with the shared secret of what it is to be a woman.

Grief touches us all in this life, it is the price of love. Some people encounter grief sooner rather than later in their lives. The death of a pet when you are a child is practice for learning about the impermanence of life and sets the tone for how we cope with loss as we go forward in the world. Many of us lose a grandparent, and eventually, our parents and we become the next generation. Sometimes we lose a sibling or a friend through accident or illness. Some take their own life and leave us in shocked silence as we contemplate the sadness that must have enveloped their soul, so absorbed in ourselves that we didn't realize their sense of hopelessness. When the order of succession is interrupted by the loss of a younger person, our world tips, and the storm of grief throws our emotional lives into chaos and confusion. When you lose a child, you lose a part of your own being, and you are never the same again. This particular grief is so profound it forever changes how you move through the world. You must learn to bear the unbearable. After

Christie died, I wanted to apologize to the people I knew who had lost a child, for thinking that as a parent I had understood their pain.

When Carrie, the founder and coordinator of the Lighthouse Book Series, asked me to write a chapter for this book, all I could think was that I didn't have anything enlightening to say; I don't have the answer to how you live with the grief of losing a child—it is the nightmare I wake to each day. It has been more than three years since Christie died, and I still feel that fight or flight response—my stomach clenching, the enormous weight in my chest, helpless and frozen. It feels like the strength I once had has vanished and my light has dimmed. I don't have the emotional stamina I once had, and in some ways, I don't even feel like the same person anymore. How could I shine a beacon of hope out in the world when I often feel like I am still groping around in the dark? What can I write that inspires another woman, another parent, to keep going when it feels like you can't, when it feels like everything is out of your control, and the decisions you are making, based on your limited experience in something so enormous, are choices between the terrible and the unthinkable? How do you keep going and find peace with the journey?

Everything now has become the before and after. Before Christie was diagnosed with leukemia, and after she died. I remember the fall of 2019. My husband, Joe, and I felt as if we were close to retirement, planning our future as empty nesters, our four children all finished post-secondary schooling and forging their paths. I wanted to start a blog, try doing more artwork, and I was thinking about when I would stop working as a realtor. We were excited to be taking time for ourselves and exploring what our lives would look like going forward. We had two big trips planned from our home on Vancouver Island that winter. The first was a motorcycle trip down the Baja with another couple, good friends that we travel well with. We came home for the holidays in December with our family and then flew to Costa Rica for the month of January 2020.

Costa Rica is where we first heard the rumors, something called the Coronavirus in China. I was baffled. The rumors continued, but we were in Central America, enjoying our long winter vacation, playing "snowbirds." I talked to the kids on the phone, especially Christie as she had just moved to Sacramento and her life was topsy-turvy with a new home, job, friends, and lots of excitement. Except, she wasn't feeling well. Her throat hurt, she said it was hard to swallow, and sometimes hard to breathe at night. She went to the doctor, blood tests were run, but nothing specific was found. Her roommate was sick too, and I suspected they had been burning the proverbial candle at both ends. Working, going out, acting like the young women in their twenties that they were.

"They say it could be mumps, Mom," she tells me. *"Or mono."*

"You can't have mumps; you were vaccinated," I say. Privately I thought, *Oh damn, I hope she doesn't have mono, that can set you back a long time.*

"They say you can still get it," she replies. She sounds worried, and she tells me her arm is swollen. *"Mom, I think I might have a blood clot."*

"You should go back to the clinic," I say, *"Get them to look again."*

She does. She takes time off work. By this time, we are home from Costa Rica and I am making plans to get rolling with real estate work and contemplating when I can fly down to see Christie. I am starting to worry more about her. She didn't come home for Christmas and has been going full steam ahead, finishing university, moving, getting a job, a place to live, and a California driver's license. I want to check in on her and see her new place in Sacramento. I am thinking Mother's Day would work for a visit, but my gut tells me I should go sooner. On February 22 she called from an ER where her roommate's dad had driven her that morning. "Mom, they took an X-ray and have done a CT scan. I have a mass in my chest. They say it is cancer."

I drop everything and fly to San Francisco, where she is being sent by ambulance, and by February 27 after a bone marrow biopsy, scans, and a surgical biopsy on the mass in her chest, we have a diagnosis: T-Cell ALL, Acute Lymphoblastic Leukemia. I remember walking into a restroom down the hall and looking at myself in the mirror, feeling numb inside. *My daughter has leukemia.* It is surreal, like I have lived this before in another life, but it is so incredibly wrong. Late that evening they moved Christie to a new unit in the hospital, as chemo needed to start immediately. As we walked slowly down the hall of the hematology-oncology unit, with the porter pushing her bed, Christie grabbed my hand and squeezed. We knew then that we were beginning a long journey. We just didn't know how it would end.

We stay in San Francisco for the induction round of chemotherapy. The aim was to hit her hard with a complex blend of chemotherapy and steroids to push her into remission with that first round. She will have more rounds of chemo, and then she will need a stem cell transplant, also known as a bone marrow transplant. She has a subtype of T-Cell ALL called Early Precursor, which is even more serious than the garden variety leukemia, as if there is such a thing. She actually does have a blood clot, and along with the mass in her chest, these things make her treatment more complex. If I had wanted to take her home right then, she would not have been able to travel. *How had she gotten so sick so fast?* Leukemia is deadly and it advances like a herd of antelope being chased by lions when unchecked.

Wrapped in the womb of the hospital, I am oblivious to the noise of the pandemic moving toward us. The first sign that it will seriously affect us is visitor restrictions. They tell us that Christie can only have one visitor per twenty-four-hour period. That means her dad, Len, and I would have to alternate twenty-four hours on and off, but I am the one who needs to spend the night with her to help with getting to the bathroom, and shower-ing. She has a peripherally inserted central catheter, a PICC line, in her groin attaching her to an IV pole, as the mass in her chest won't allow for one near her collarbone, where it is easier to manage bathing. Her dad wants to be with her as much as I do, but she is a young woman and wants her mom for personal care. My husband, Joe, Christie's stepdad for twenty-three years, needing to feel purposeful, has brought his truck down from Canada and he leaves with all her belongings packed up into the back of it, after retrieving them from Sacramento. At first, Christie had protested. She wanted to keep her place with her friends, but I can see months of treatment ahead, and no reason to keep renting a room in a house two hours from the hospital. She is just beginning to process all the things she will lose. Her health, her home, her job, her independence, her hair, her fertility. Our minds can't possibly go to the next step, the possibility of losing her life. It is unthinkable. Her dad, having flown down when I did, takes her car loaded with the last of her belongings back to Canada. We know now that her student medical plan will cover this hospital stay, but will not cover a bone marrow transplant, and we will be returning to Canada. I am actually relieved, and after speak-ing with our family doctor at home, I am reassured that her treatment in Vancouver will be on par with anywhere in the world.

By the time we are ready to leave the hospital in San Francisco, after a full month of intensive treatment, the world has shut down. All visitors have been asked to leave the hospital but thankfully I am given grace, and they allow me to stay in with Christie, as long as I don't leave the building. We board a near-empty plane, masked and unsure, having paid for business class tickets, but there really wasn't any need. It was eerily empty and silent, and we arrive in Vancouver with a minimum of fanfare, whisked through the airport in a wheelchair, and over to Nanaimo. I was desperately relieved to be home, even if only for a day.

We have about thirty-six hours at home before meeting with the oncologist in Vancouver on Monday. That is when we are told we must find a place to live within thirty minutes of the hospital. Treatment starts Wednesday with a PET scan, and she will need a new Hickman line surgically implanted in her chest to begin the next round of chemo. I wasn't anticipating that. I thought we would go back and forth to the mainland for treatment and return home, perhaps even having some chemo locally. *No*, they say. It is a specialized treatment, and she needs to be at the Bone Marrow Transplant Unit. She will need to stay in Vancouver for several months leading up to her transplant and for one hundred days afterward. The enormity of what we are facing is beginning to take hold and I am overwhelmed, but I try to remain calm so that Christie feels more secure. She is already emotional from the steroids she is on, not to mention the trauma of the situation, and the stress is taking a toll. My husband, Joe, finds us an apartment in Yaletown. It is furnished and bright on the twenty-seventh floor, with a small balcony overlooking False Creek. Christie's bedroom looks down on the lights of a hotel across the street, where they have lit up their vacant rooms in the shape of a giant heart. BC Place Stadium lights twinkle nearby, and my room looks over the old Expo '86 site towards Science World. The streets are quiet, and each evening at seven the people in the nearby apartment buildings come out to clap and generally make a cacophony of noise in support of health workers in the pandemic.

In the face of leukemia treatment, we are so fortunate to have this tiny oasis in the city. I can walk to the grocery store in one direction, and to Costco in another, where I pick up prescriptions to fill the daily pill containers with a mind-boggling plethora of medications. It takes us about twelve minutes to go down the elevator, into the car, and across the Cambie Street bridge to Vancouver General Hospital, where I drop Christie off at the doors each day to go into the Leukemia/Bone Marrow Transplant Daycare unit alone. She has her second round of chemo, and her blood counts are monitored continually. Platelets, neutrophils, and red blood cells are counted. I am learning a new language of medical terms. Her third round of chemo requires five days as an "in-patient." It will be her first taste of in-patient hospitalization in Canada.

"*The food is horrible, Mom*," she groans.

With the steroids Christie is on to help battle her leukemia, she is ravenously hungry, despite the rounds of chemo being pumped into her body. Back in San Francisco, the food was ordered from a menu that reminded me of a "Ricky's" restaurant, and you could have pretty much anything you wanted. I tried once in Vancouver to send food in with her, but with Covid regulations, she was reprimanded by the nurse. The pandemic restrictions were relentless. One day, she was sobbing when I picked her up outside the hospital. In the daycare unit, there are "chair rooms," which are shared areas for patients to receive medications, chemo, and fluids, and wait for consultations. She had begun to make a tenuous friendship with another fellow there named Evan, who looked to be in his twenties as well. They had chatted, commiserating about having cancer as a young adult, in this place with a mostly geriatric population. A doctor was speaking with him, going over test results, and explained to him that he had relapsed, that his cancer was back and he was dying. He was devastated, and alone, without family for support. They may have been adults, but these were our *children*. It was terrifying and heralded a point where we began to realize that this could also be Christie's fate. And yet, we still had so much hope.

The spring melds into summer, and we watch seagulls nesting on the tops of buildings from our apartment, and people with their dogs in the park below our balcony. When I finally take Christie in for her bone marrow transplant on July 2, loaded down with a suitcase full of cards and well wishes, her own pillows and blankets and snacks for an anticipated month alone in the hospital, I go home to the island. We FaceTime each day, multiple times, but it is agony watching her undergo this most difficult treatment by herself. She is frightened but so very brave and determined. She wants it to be over, and to carry on with her life, even one that she cannot yet foresee. The loss of fertility due to the chemotherapy and radiation is a hard pill for her to swallow, and it weighs heavily on her. We talk of her future, adoption, and in-vitro fertilization with donor eggs, but she is devastated, and as a mom, I feel her pain acutely.

I have flashbacks of her bravery through her fear. I remember her calling me in the night during the radiation treatments. They were the hardest, as she knew that at this point if her ovaries weren't finished off from the chemo, the radiation would do it. Her isolation, living within the world of the bone marrow transplant unit was surreal. She sent us a fast-forward video of her twenty-minute stretcher ride from her room on floor T15, underground through a maze of industrial-looking hallways, to the radiation center. From her vantage point, we can see the new slippers bought for her hospital stay framing the view of her route. She tells me how she couldn't stop crying on the first day of radiation, the technician stopping to calm her; on the second day she saw a young mom there with her little boy, about four or five years old, and she was sorry for how sad and exhausted the mom looked. It was typical of her to be concerned and sad for someone else. The third day pushed her hard against a wall of tolerance, but she kept her eyes on the goal, and she made it through. It was six days of myeloablative conditioning before the transplant, three of hard chemotherapy, and three of radiation. Her own stem cells had been decimated, and clinging to life, the bags of precious cells from her unknown, anonymous donor are fed through her line, and the waiting begins.

In the following days, we excitedly count platelets, neutrophils, and red blood cells produced by her newly engrafted stem cells. Her blood type has changed from B positive to O positive. It feels like a miracle and we are so thankful for this gift from a stranger in the middle of a global pandemic. She is released after twenty-six days in hospital, but she has a long way to go.

I look back on those hard days post-transplant and see Christie walking into the hospital in her checkered Vans, wearing her favorite pink ball cap, carrying a backpack with her iPad and snacks slung over her shoulder, sometimes shuffling into the hospital in exhaustion, neuropathy in her feet. There were times I had to take her up to the unit in a wheelchair and leave her there. Once she had an infection, Epstein Barr Virus resurfaced from somewhere in her body, and she was devastated to be hospitalized for another few weeks, alone again. I hated it so much, this separation, this aspect of leukemia in the time of Covid. It added so much to the complexity of treatment, to the pressure of it all, as if it wasn't enough already. The Covid pandemic was yet another piece that added so much weight to her treatment. For myself, I had to face my own need to be needed, and reconcile being a caregiver who often couldn't provide care. Sandwiched between fear and hope, I had to be strong for Christie.

During these months of treatment that Christie and I spent in Vancouver, when she was an out-patient and I couldn't accompany her into the hospital due to Covid regulations, I would drop her off for blood work and appointments, and then walk or bike along Vancouver's seawall, feeling the gift of fresh air, flowers, birds, and sunshine. I would pick up her favorite bagels with cream cheese at Granville Island, go to the grocery store, and try to spend some time feeding my tired soul. When she wasn't in the hospital we would do things together that made her feel better. Once we went to the aquarium together, masked and by appointment so that we could be separate from other people. I have a photo of us on the seawall in Stanley Park when she felt well enough to take a walk. I had art supplies at the condo, and we binge-watched Netflix: The World's Toughest Race, Survivor, and more. I read a few books, but my concentration has been poor since her diagnosis, and still hasn't fully recovered. Later, I read Suleika Jaouad's memoir, *Between Two Kingdoms,* and it helped me better understand the perspective of a young woman undergoing leukemia treatment. I long for that time again, and despite the circumstances, I am grateful that we had those months together.

We finally came home in October and celebrated her one hundred days post-transplant. It was a huge milestone, but what we didn't realize was that in the aftermath of her transplant, we were only at the beginning of her healing. We made it through the rest of the fall and Christmas, with some beautiful times, but also with family strife amplified in ways we could not have imagined. I wish we could say we were the picture-perfect family, happy and relieved to be out of arm's reach of the hospital, but it was emotional and challenging. I wish it had been different, better. I hang tightly to the phrase given to me by my wise step-daughter Jess: *If it could have been different, it would have been,* and I have to believe that we did our best.

I remember the oncologist telling Christie her leukemia had relapsed. It was February 22, 2021, one year to the day she had first been told she had cancer. I was downstairs, outside the hospital, listening to her appointment on the phone, Christie alone in his office. He told her that her most recent blood work had shown her leukemia was back, and that any treatment would be palliative, not curative. I still feel like I have nails in my stomach from that moment. Our options were few, he said they could try Nelarabine, a new type of chemotherapy, and do some radiation to reduce the mass in her chest that had grown again. She came down the elevator alone, collapsing into my arms sobbing. In the coming days, we struggled through more phone conferences, Christie angry and devastated, all of us shell-shocked. Her romantic friend from the USA, Howie, arrived. He quarantined, and they got married on our patio. I don't think he really understood the gravity of the situation, but I have to give him credit for showing up, for being what she needed at that time. They had a weekend honeymoon in Victoria after her last radiation treatment.

Christie began researching other hospitals, and finally, after the round of chemo in Vancouver failed to stop her leukemia from advancing, she said she wanted to try going to MD Anderson Cancer Center in Houston, Texas. Her oncologist in Vancouver reassured her that if she went, she could still come back and would always be their patient as well. The doctor said that he had worked at MD Anderson, and said they would most likely have something they could try there that wasn't available here, but it would not be curative. He was kind but did not offer false hope. I was afraid she would spend her last weeks of life alone, and then die in a Texas hospital. We were all in agony. She was angry with me for not being on board right away, and in hindsight, I don't blame her. I wanted her to have peace; she wanted hope.

Christie did go to Houston, and I had to let her have that time with Howie, although she spent the first month alone in the hospital down there, still under Covid regulations. I followed a few weeks later to be with her, and we settled in for the second round of chemo. Finally, I was allowed to go into the hospital after speaking with her oncologist, who seemed to think that if Christie could get into remission, a second transplant would give her about a ten percent chance of life. But she needed to be in remission first and there were significant leukemia blasts present and fluid on her lungs. Ten days after they administered a second round of brutal chemo, she was admitted for the excruciating headache pain she was in after having a lumbar puncture, and her blood counts had plummeted. Her heart rate went up and her blood pressure dropped. In the early morning hours of the ICU, they drained fluid from her heart and intubated her. The volume of chemo was too toxic, and her organs were failing, but she had been willing to risk everything to live. I can't imagine how much courage it must have taken for Christie to walk into that hospital and undergo more devastating treatment with everything she had been through already.

She died that day, on a Wednesday in June; Howie and I were with her. I have agonized over all of it, rolling it around in my head, continually, day after day ever since. I want to go back and try again, to see if I can change something, anything. Sometimes there's just no opportunity for peace, in life or in death.

We were helpless in the face of leukemia, but Christie refused to back down. She fought like the lion she was, hoping for more time, more opportunity for love, for a family of her own. Her life had blazed fiercely, and our whole family feels the absence of her flame. We had to stand by and watch. Our attempts at helping her find peace were rejected as she raged, and waged a war that ultimately, in her own way, she won. She didn't live, but death would not take her spirit, and she walks in light now, stopping by to touch us often, to remind us of who she was. Her spirit, her energy, while she is no longer with us among the living, is vibrating in a way that I feel as a gentle touch on my shoulder when she is near. I think over there in the beyond, she has found the peace that eluded her here.

I woke up once in the night, in the months after she died, and went outside to look at the sky. The stars were shining so brightly I felt as if Christie was looking down at me. In the morning, when I woke, the sky was clear blue, not a star to be found, but I knew they were still there, out in the universe, shining with all their might. I know Christie is out there too; but like the stars, I can't see her, and her absence fills me with a longing so intense that I have to breathe deeply and hold myself still, the need to hug her, talk with her again unfulfilled. My mind reviews all the mistakes I made as a parent and I want a "do-over" so that I can try to get it right this time, to do a better job. I want to shield her from the hard knocks she had, find a way to be kinder, more understanding, more supportive. My mother used to say that hindsight is twenty-twenty, and she was right, but even with hindsight, I know I couldn't have saved her from all of it. I am only human, as Christie would have said, and we aren't meant to lead perfect lives. I want to forgive myself for not being able to shield her from everything that life threw at her, especially, ultimately, leukemia. Forgiveness. That is one of the things I learned from my beautiful girl. She could be fierce and angry, but she forgave freely.

I try to remember the simple, happy moments, and I wish I had more photos. I envy the moms of today who take photos on their cell phones by the hundreds and thousands. I rely on snapshots from poor cameras, developed and printed, faded in albums or in a box, negatives lost. I relish stories from people who knew her. They are among my greatest treasures, those few stories people have shared with me of their memories of Christie. Since I rely so heavily on my own memories, and there are parts of her life that I wasn't present for: in university, her travels, even from high school, I long to hear more about my daughter from the people she touched in her life. I live and pray for the occasional visits she makes to my dreams. Once, I was able to hug her, and another time she walked into the kitchen, laughing. It seemed she had managed this brief visit, to tell me she was happy. Sometimes she has come to me as a child, and others as an adult. I wake up feeling lost, searching for details, wanting to return to the dream, just to see her again.

When I hear of other people beginning a journey like ours, my heart pounds and my chest constricts as I remember the early days with compassion. There is no way out, only through, and I ache to think that someone else is facing their version of a cancer pathway with their child.

An actual journey and the metaphorical one feel as if they should be reflected in one another. In the fall, four months after Christie died, Joe and I traveled to the island of Crete. The ancient world there is closer, and the dead walk beside you in the ruins. I move through the world differently now, and although at times I feel disconnected, the travel shifts something in me and creates some motion. I think of her and wonder if she is watching all the time. I look for signs that she is near, even when I am far from home.

I feel Christie in the light that is shining on the ocean, through the windows in the morning and evening, and in the rosy glow reflected on the mountains as the sun sets. I feel her nearby as I write in my journal or work with paint and collage. After coming home from her transplant, Christie declared herself an artist and started painting with resin and acrylic. She was like that, just putting herself out there, into the role of what she wanted to be, manifesting by announcing it. I still have her blog transcripts written in the early days of her diagnosis and treatment. It is another part of her that resonates, that I can learn from.

I've learned from Christie not to wait to write or paint or start something until you think you are ready. The only time is now. Each day becomes a work of art. Sometimes I am in the "messy middle," where nothing is working and all I want to do is lie down and sleep for a year. I realize that if I am going to survive, I need to create a life with purpose again. This is, in itself, an act of creativity; finding a balance between going through the mundane aspects of life: cooking, cleaning, shopping, and being in a place of positivity and movement. In the three years since Christie died, I have learned to take better care of myself, to be grateful for simple things, and allow myself to be soothed by the peace that is in the moment. I bake cookies and bread. Christie loved to bake. Her best friend Shannon and I joked that it was her love language, to bake dozens of cookies and give them away. She taught us all to be kind, and generous. It is in these small creative acts that I find a way forward, towards a light that shines through the darkness.

Christie taught me compassion. Amidst her own pain and fear, she was devastated because she didn't want us to be the family whose daughter died from leukemia. Today, I find compassion in a hug, or words from a friend, especially those who have known grief. I go to the support group, The Compassionate Friends, and find companionship with the other parents who have lost children. It is a strange sort of sorority. While the group isn't restricted to mothers, we are the ones who gather and light candles beside the photos of our lost children, sharing the weight of our grief. It provides a place where I don't feel like an outsider, as I sometimes do around other women. I still want to talk about Christie, but not everyone is comfortable hearing about your dead child. I think it reminds them of their own vulnerability and a place they never want to visit. While I really do want to hear about their families, the kids graduating, getting married, and having babies, I still feel a pang for the life Christie didn't get to lead. Only those people closest to me, who also know grief in one form or another, seem to understand, and I am grateful for them.

I try meditation, but I procrastinate and fidget, climbing on and off my mental hamster wheel, so my morning walk near the beach and through our woodland trails becomes my meditation. Yoga helps me feel grounded, too, and as I intermittently commit to a regular practice, it is a good enough reason to travel to an island in Greece for a retreat with my best friend and stepsister. It is a place out of time, and the energy is layered with so many lifetimes, that I find a little more movement. I have tried other more spiritual and energetic therapies: Reiki, and sound baths, and I visited a medium a few months after Christie died, the longing to connect and speak with my daughter visceral. I want to ask forgiveness, for being alive when she faced death. I want her back.

There is no magical way through grief; perhaps we remain in that dark land forever, learning to practice living with a rich fullness within the spectrum of light we are given in this lifetime. As time goes on, and we work at healing, more sunlight shines on us, and we begin to recognize landmarks, to know joy again, allowing space for grief alongside joy, peace and contentment. I do think there is magic in simple rituals: a daily walk, a nap, a lunch date, a chat with one of my beautiful living children, or a good friend. I am grateful for my relationship with my husband, our kids, their spouses, our family and friends, for a snuggle with our grandbaby, who brings joy and laughter and new life back to all of us, and the assurance that there will be more. There is the taking care of oneself as if you were the child, not the parent or caregiver. In this caregiving and connection, I suppose I find some redemption for what couldn't be. This story is still emerging, and I don't have all the answers, most particularly because we all have our own journey. My version of this will be different from what Christie's story was, and that of her siblings, her friends, and her other parents. I can only walk my own path and tell my own story, but along the way, I light candles for Christie and for those who walk through this darkness on paths of their own making, in hopes that they will find light along the way.

We shake with joy, we shake with grief. What a time they have, these two housed as they are in the same body. - Mary Oliver

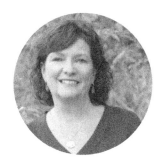

MARNIE LAW

Marnie Law lives in Nanoose Bay on Vancouver Island with her husband Joe. Having lived on the island her whole life, she is steeped in the lifestyle here and raised her family with a love of both home and travel. She loves the beaches and walking trails, and can be found swimming in the ocean when summer arrives. Marnie recently started writing on Substack under "The Leo Art Collective" and can be reached directly at marnielaw@shaw.ca. She loves listening to music and podcasts, art, reading, traveling, and spending time with her family.

Photo credit: Erin Edwards

Everything she touches becomes illuminated and changed for the better.

CHAPTER FIVE

The Little Alchemist MagicK

Written by Gwen Haas

This story is about a little girl who lost her magicK. This story is about how this little girl remembered that life is full of magicK and mystery and wonder and awe, and that life doesn't have to be confusing or scary. Life is a weaving of a tapestry where each thread holds a story, a message, a lesson, that we as a collective are moving through this existence. We are so much more connected than we even realize we are. In this very moment in time we are playing out, moving through, healing, and shifting—honoring those who have come before us and those who will come after us, knowing that every decision we make, every path we take, every act we move into, is in fact creating a ripple of effect forwards and backwards in time.

I call the little girl who lost her magicK my little alchemist. Throughout this story, I am spelling magicK with a K, because this little girl inside of me wants to put her special mark in this story and she spells it with a K. In this way, I feel like I am re-owning and giving voice to the magicKal part of myself that this story is all about. I am this little girl, my own little alchemist, and she is me.

And I do believe that you picked up this book and are reading these words at this time in your life for a reason. I believe that there are guides and teachers that come to help awaken our gifts, our senses, our awarenesses—to help us move through our traumas, to heal those wounds that we may, at first glance, think happened in this lifetime, but may be an echo from our ancestor's past.

And there is an opportunity for us to shift it, to heal it, and ultimately to remember our magicK. Everyone has their own definition of magicK, as they should, but for me, the magicK is in the dance and the merging of the unseen world into the physical realms. It is in the beautiful synchronicities that happen without even asking, or even more delicious, is when I pray for something and it shows up in all its glory, more Divine and breathing-taking than I could have ever imagined on my own. It's when my heart feels like it is being kissed by the Divine. This is part of the alchemy of magicK that has the potential to rise within us all. From all green lights on my drive to an appointment to feeling a warm breeze kiss my cheek at the perfect time when I'm talking with a loved one that has crossed over. I believe that so many of us have lost touch with our magicK in this lifetime; whether that is from protecting parts of ourselves that could not be recognized in our environment so we shut those magicKal parts of ourselves down to survive, or if it's from past traumas that may feel too great to dive into or be aware of at this time. Yet as we start to move through the healing process, we become awakened to hidden loss and grief that had laid dormant until now, but ultimately there will come a remembering of all the magicK that is within us and always has been. This coming into contact with our magicK once again is like remembering a part of ourselves that has gone missing—it is like finding a lost piece of the puzzle of our being.

MagicK has been in my life for the last twenty-one years. When I was thirty-one years old, I experienced a Kundalini awakening, where the gifts of being a seer awakened within me. It happened during my first experience with meditation with a spiritual teacher. It was such a profound experience, and I barely have words to describe it. It was as if I was surfing through the universe and being shown the vastness of life and all of creation. As I was moving through this experience the teacher cradled my head in his hands and helped to keep me grounded in my physical body, otherwise, I felt like I might sail away in the vastness. From this point forward, I began having two different levels of awareness unfolding at the same time within me. I began to witness the non-ordinary world, or unseen world, weaving into the ordinary physical realm. My life began to feel more magicKal from this moment on. The gifts that arose from this awakening in me ranged from receiving a subtle flow of information from all of creation, nature speaking to me, to having all manner of visions that helped me to comprehend the totality of different and complex situations and not become lost in the issues. It also sparked inner knowings, premonitions, and channeling of Divine healing energies, through myself and for the benefit of others. As the years went on, more abilities and gifts would enter my life related to this initial opening. The experience of seeing the extraordinary has become my ordinary, everyday experience. As I progressed on my healing journey, through many peaks and valleys, more and more would be revealed to me, until finally, a little girl emerged from within me that was full of innocent magicK and alchemy. Everything she touches became illuminated and changed for the better.

This magicKal journey led me on a path to begin cultivating a safe environment within myself that would become a welcoming home to the little alchemist within me. As my safety grew, this little alchemist began to emerge, *or shall I say return to me?* Through this healing work, I began to feel like I was coming together, like pieces of a puzzle falling back into place. As an adult, it took me a long time to feel safe inside my body. This young part of myself lived most of her life deeply confused by the world that surrounded her. She was highly sensitive, and because of this, her nervous system was constantly processing large amounts of information in each interaction with the world. But she didn't know this. All that she knew was how to hide her magicKal self away from the world that felt so full of pain and suffering. It would take a long time to make room for my stressed and fried nervous system to unravel without making myself go sideways and getting lost in the sensations and emotions that were arising within me. It took a lot of re-learning and work to create a safe nurturing environment, especially since it wasn't my childhood experience when I was growing up. My normal baseline consisted of the fight/flight response, so this involved a re-learning and an experiencing of something new for my system. Slowly, I was teaching my nervous system a different way to be.

During a session with my teacher, who was guiding me through a healing practice where she asked me to sink into the ground like I was growing roots into the earth, she cued me to imagine the soil of a garden that had just been freshly tilled. I could feel the soft soil between my toes as I sank my feet down into the welcoming earth.

As soon as I began to grow roots into the ground, I received a vision of trees in a garden. This garden was consumed with weeds, the soil felt sparse and depleted and filled with emptiness. I could feel dysfunction oozing like a pus-filled wound, but the trees that surrounded this garden had me at "Hello." The trees wrapped the garden and layered themselves in a way that made me feel safe, like I was being held in a community, and had this unwavering presence that was steadfast and always watching over me. The trees felt abundantly ALIVE to me. They felt wise, ancient, and very familiar, like a circle of wise elders from my ancestral past. Luckily for me, my teacher was very responsive to my visions and gave me space to allow them to guide the growth of supporting energies in my garden that would later become resources that I would call forth every time I brought a hurt part of myself to the garden to heal.

With every session, as traumas came up, my teacher encouraged me to take my frozen traumatized parts to my garden for some healing. As each part healed they would transform back into their original essence. Each time I experienced this restoration, I felt the alchemy of processing unfolding within me; the act of changing one substance into another. In this case it was the hurt parts of myself that had been damaged through earlier wounding being restored to their original form and brilliance, playing out as the alchemical process. I may not have fully realized it at the time, but the restoration of all of these parts inside of me, were like the puzzle pieces coming back together and ultimately they formed what I now call the little alchemist within me. This is the part of me that can process and create transformation when needed, guide me on my path, and open my eyes to a more magicKal life.

The tending to my visualized garden didn't come easily. This involved digging and cultivating the depleted soil. The more fertile soil I created through this process, the more new ground it gave me to host more of the lost parts of myself that emerged for healing and integration. I remember pulling an overwhelming amount of weeds with roots that felt like they were unending. With every trauma came its own area of weeds that seemed to blind me to the weeding that had already been accomplished. But over time, as I cleared the weeds and cultivated the soil, something happened. I started to see and sense the dark richness of the soil. The lush, rich soil had this tantalizing smell that invoked this deep, sacred, unwavering presence within me. My heart, like the trees, felt ALIVE and it felt like the sun was rising once again in my heart. Joy had returned to the home of my being. Throughout the years more magicKal experiences would unfold with each piece of healing work that I did in my garden. It made sense that my little alchemist would feel ready to be seen in this environment. That which once felt unsettled, uncertain, and disturbed within me, now felt safe, nourished, and nurtured in this environment.

The ground is now rich and abundant and able to process and digest all that I bring into the space and creates something much more beneficial for my highest good. It's the kind of environment where a child can be a child. Where they can be anywhere in the house and play and feel safe knowing that their parents are close by, and they'll be okay. It's a place to be safe to play, explore, and be curious, like all children naturally are.

Over the last few years, I've had many resources grow roots and blossom in my garden. It's not just plants that live in my garden but animals as well. It's a whole ecosystem! For instance, now when I ground into the earth, I am met by the network of mycelium found beneath the surface that eagerly greets me like long lost cousins. This chain of cousins have become one of the strongest super powers in my garden. They can digest everything and anything, like maggots cleaning a wound and exposing fresh, new potential. Going into this next layer of the earth, past the mycelium, I hear my grandmother calling me in her Polish accent, "Gwendia, Gwendia, come eat, come eat!" She is wanting to replenish me with healthy nutrients, minerals, and deep ancient wisdom from the lineage of our elders that came before us. I also have this adorable white baby calf that came to me one day and has been with me since. It would frolic around and was always available to regulate any parts of myself that I brought into my garden. I always know a piece of healing work is complete when the hurt part within me that I was working with runs off to play with the baby calf. By nurturing and growing my inner garden, healing these deep wounds that laid dormant inside of me, I birthed a new space within me that my little alchemist finally felt safe enough to come home to.

I felt like it was from this new healthy space that my little alchemist started to emerge in a new and surprising way for me. I'm a highly sensitive person, so I was referred to this naturopath that specializes in more complex and unusual combinations of signs and symptoms. She works with electrodermal testing and for a highly sensitive soul, as myself, this machine resonated deeply with me. It works with frequencies and gauges imbalances within the body. I'm sure most wouldn't find this fascinating but for me, it connects with my gifts and abilities of being a seer whose entire world is connected and intertwined with frequencies and within balances and imbalances. For myself, the dance is a constant in real time, meaning when things are off, I sense it immediately and my whole ecosystem works to bring it back into balance, which can be most uncomfortable at times. I felt seen and like my inner workings felt understood by this machine. It's like it put my inner experience into a language that could be heard by the naturopath and others, as if the machine was a bridge between us. Finally, the indescribable inside of me had words and someone was able to understand my language. My first visit with the naturopath was when I noticed my little alchemist differently. This is where I began to feel her begin to express herself outside of my inner world and garden and into the external world.

On my first visit to the naturopath, it was an ordinary drive from my house to the office, nothing unusual happened. I wasn't nervous going into the appointment and I had a great connection with the ladies at the front desk which was a good sign for me and gave me reassurance that I was on the right path seeking help here. I went into the naturopath's office, and she smiled and asked where I would like to start. Out of nowhere, these intense, frantic feelings of fear surged through my body and before I knew what was happening I was telling the naturopath about an extremely traumatic time in my life. I was overcome with strong emotion at that moment. I was snot-crying and a vision was arising in my mind's eye. The next thing I knew I was dangling my fingers in front of my face to describe the vision to the naturopath. It was like my hand was my nervous system and my fingers were the fried wires. I kept hearing the word, "fried," being said in my mind.

You'd think at this point one would be mortified, but nope. I heard myself tell the naturopath that I was acutely aware that I was unable to make eye contact with her, as there was so much shame coursing through my body at the moment. This was my little alchemist arising in me. She was bringing this undigested experience of previously stuck emotion up to the surface to be processed in this safe environment. This was significant because this was an external environment, rather than my inner garden. Part of the way the magicK was arising for me at this moment, was that I was now finding exterior environments that were a reflection of the safety I had cultivated within my inner garden. This is both a sign of healing and an example of alchemy at work.

When a trauma arises within me and is ready for release, all of what is stuck within that frozen space comes bubbling into my awareness. In this case, I was feeling deep shame, so much so that I couldn't make eye contact and fear was coursing through me, as this blind-siding event of huge emotion and vision suddenly blurted, seemingly out of nowhere, into my experience. These are all of the ways how my body speaks to me and how I receive information. This would be the uncomfortable part of my process when I meet the imbalances within myself and it adds an entire new layer to the phrase, lean into your wounds. Although this had been a huge emotional event in the naturopath's office, I could feel how the little alchemist within me had been the one to push all of these feelings towards the surface, guiding me into processing it, because she could feel that she was safe here. This is a big part of how she communicates with me and works her magicK through me.

I wouldn't witness or experience my little alchemist communicating again until my next naturopathic appointment three months later. By the second visit, I was very aware that my little alchemist had chosen this naturopath, and oddly enough, the naturopath didn't think I was crazy after all that had unfolded in the first visit. I felt like my little alchemist loved this naturopath at first glance, for her wildly curly, untamed hair that spoke to the free child part of me. By now, she was becoming comfortable with showing herself to me in the world, but only when the environment felt safe. I felt like this was her sensing and knowing when the space was free of judgment or fear, and the environment was open to whatever arose. Over time, she would continue to show herself more and more to me, and that is where the book, *The Me I Didn't See*, came into place.

I felt like the title of this book really was speaking to me. Coming online within myself was the me that I didn't even see for much of my life, which I now understand is my little alchemist. I was randomly scrolling in this Women Over 50 in Alberta Facebook group, when I came across this post of a book titled, *The Me I Didn't See,* which is the predecessor to the book you're reading now. It was the little alchemist within me that screamed for joy and nudged me towards the title.

It was an immediate connection to the title of the book. I had no idea what the book was even about, all I knew for certain was that it stirred something deeply within me. It felt as if that depleted void, that longing, and that yearning inside of me was experiencing a taste of some nourishment. I wondered to myself, "Could it possibly be; that long, lost part inside of me—the me I didn't see?" I believe this was my little alchemist pushing me towards this book, as if there was more of her to see and discover. I truly believe in fate, in life's magicK. I believe when we are in flow, life is magicK and when we are not in flow, this is an opportunity for growth. As Rumi, my favorite Sufi philosopher quotes, "The wound is the place where light enters you." My little alchemist was adamant that I pursue sharing my story in this book. Without even thinking about it, I reached out to the person who had posted about *The Me I Didn't See* on Facebook. They then introduced me to Carrie who is the creator of The Lighthouse Project, and here we are! I'm here, writing a story about how I began to experience the little alchemist within me and giving a voice to that part of myself in a really big and external way. The fear and resistance to writing my story that arose inside of me didn't have a chance to stop me. I could feel my little alchemist coming out again during that conversation with Carrie. I felt her scanning Carrie as we spoke about the details of how to become a co-author in this book. I felt her curiosity and excitement as Carrie described how writing a chapter and becoming a part of the Lighthouse Project actually worked.

Then as I was sharing with Carrie about myself and the story that I wanted to tell in this book, something interesting happened inside of me. I felt my little alchemist expanding and growing inside of me, so much so, that she was almost touching my skin. It was like she was reclaiming her space within me. I stopped and closed my eyes to savor the moment. This was a beautiful integration piece, and I am now able to embody more of the free child, magicKal, and alchemist-like qualities in my life. It's a practice, and I am by no means perfect, but I now hear my little alchemist more clearly and feel her nudges more fully in my everyday life.

And so, I am grateful that this little alchemist inside of me, who was the me I didn't see for many years of my life, has come back to open me up to curiosity, to help me to see the world in new ways, and to guide me even deeper on my journey of healing. It was as if she was this weaver of magicK, this alchemist this entire time and I just didn't know it was her yet.

Each of us has a little alchemist inside of us who is waiting for us to come into a place and a space in our life where we can have the ability to weave one's magicK through life, and to remember the magicK that was there all along.

By nurturing and growing my inner garden, healing these deep wounds that laid dormant inside of me, I birthed a new space within me that my little alchemist finally felt safe enough to come home to and make itself known in the outer world. It's in this environment where the magicK within each of us begins to unfold, and the little alchemist inside all of us can begin to emerge in our everyday life.

May each one of us have the courage to heal the wounds of our past and reunite with our little alchemist within so that we become the weaver of our own alchemy in this lifetime, creating ripple effects of blessings and nourishment to all those that have come before us and those that will come after us.

Many Blessings

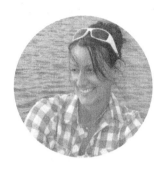

GWEN HAAS

Gwen Haas is known for her insatiable curiosity, love of getting to know others, and the ability to make people feel seen and comfortable.

Gwen has an immense love of the mystical in her life and feels drawn to everything in that realm. She enjoys working with all of her gifts and abilities using them to be in service of others' highest good.

In her spare time, she enjoys classes in spirituality and mysticism, chant circles, community dream circles, philosophical conversations, poetry, markets, and quaint coffee shops with a good book. Gwen enjoys spending time with her elderly mother, her three children, five grandchildren, and three grand dogs. Her grandchildren teach her in each moment to connect with the playfulness and freedom of her inner child. It's through her grandchildren that she is able to witness how the effect of the healing work that she has integrated trickles down through the family lineage creating a new seed of possibility to blossom in the newer generations.

She would love to connect with any readers who are curious and wanting to dive deeper into themselves. Gwen can be reached at Gwenseerofthesoul@gmail.com.

It wasn't the biggest, most obvious moment that brought me down, it was the one I didn't see coming, the one that caused everything to fall apart.

Sensitivity Advisory: This chapter references personal experiences of chronic illness, medical assistance in dying (MAiD), and PTSD.

CHAPTER SIX

A Lifetime of Shame

Written by Erin Gorrie

The room was dimly lit, barely cutting through the haze of cigarette smoke. A beautiful, confident woman on stage moved to the slow, hypnotic beat of the music, commanding the attention of every single man in the room. To my seventeen year old self, this was glamor—bold, beautiful women, mysterious shadows, and a room charged with something I couldn't quite describe but desperately wanted to be part of. So when the door to that life opened for me, I walked right in without a second thought.

Back then, when you did a private dance, you stood on a small box right in front of the man, out in the open for everyone to see. Nobody dared to touch you, bouncers would jump on anyone who tried. I had just finished one of those dances. I picked up the box and turned to walk away, and I froze. There he was. My dad. He was standing there, his piercing blue eyes locking onto mine. The shame hit me like a wave. I didn't know what to do, so I blurted out, "What are you doing here?"

His response was ice-cold, no emotion in his voice. "What are *you* doing here?" The emphasis on "you" sent me reeling. It wasn't just a question. It was a judgment. In that moment, I felt small, dirty, ashamed. I dropped the box and ran upstairs to the dressing room.

In the dressing room, the other girls could see it in my face—something was horribly wrong. One of them grabbed my arm, asking what happened. "My dad's here," I said, the words barely escaping before I burst into tears. Panic began to set in. "What now? What do I do?" I felt trapped, like my world was closing in on me. I could hear my dad identifying himself as a police officer confronting the owner. His words growing louder, angrier. I heard him say "Do you know how old she is?" My heart sank. I thought, "This is it. He's going to drag me out of here. I'm never coming back." The humiliation was unbearable. Instinctively, the girls rushed to help me, packing up my things, offering words of comfort. But I couldn't focus. One of the girls led me out the back door where my boyfriend was waiting. He had seen everything unfold. We quickly jumped into his car, my hands trembling as we sped away. As we drove, I was sure my dad was following us. I couldn't shake the feeling of dread. We drove an hour to my boyfriend's house, but I couldn't sleep that night. My mind raced, knowing my life had changed forever.

I was born the oldest of two girls. My sister was born exactly one year after me, on my first birthday, and from that day on, I never knew a world without her. My dad was a new police officer when I was born. He'd been at the police college while my mom was pregnant with me. By the time my sister came along, he was already deep into his career, which meant that, for the most part, my mom raised us. She was a stay-at-home mom back then, and everything she did revolved around us.

As my dad's career progressed, we moved a few times to different small towns in the province. When I was six, he was transferred to Northwestern Ontario, and that's where my life took a turn I never could have predicted. At ten, my mom was diagnosed with chronic progressive multiple sclerosis. It was 1985, and back then, no one really knew what MS was. My sister and I thought she was dying. No one explained her diagnosis to us properly. All we knew was that people who got really sick usually had cancer and died, so in our minds, that meant she was dying. Even though we were reassured otherwise, that fear stayed with us.

Those early years were a blur of figure skating, Girl Guides, gymnastics, waterskiing, and growing up in each other's shadow. My sister and I were inseparable, as were our identities. Our mom dressed us alike, we played the same sports, had the same friends, it was like we were twins. My mom's battle with the disease consumed her, and in many ways, my sister and I slipped into the background.

We moved again before high school, this time closer to Toronto for my mom's treatment. It was around then that I began to crave attention—particularly from boys. I felt desperate to be seen. That desperation only grew as I approached seventeen—the summer that changed everything.

That summer, I took a job at my aunt and uncle's home on the outskirts of Toronto babysitting my cousins during the week. But what I was really doing in the evenings and on weekends became a secret I carefully guarded.

That first night, after my friend and I spotted the ad for exotic dancers in the local paper, I felt my world shift in ways I never expected. Stepping into the bar was like entering another universe, one where the air was thick with smoke and secrets. Surrounded by the bar's dim lighting, the bright stage lights stood out, making the whole place feel irresistibly glamorous. The pounding bass of the music echoed through my body, and the whispers of men's voices created an undercurrent of something electric. Everything felt so far from the small-town life I had known, the dark, the flashing lights, the haze of cigarette smoke swirling with possibility. It felt like freedom.

The owner barely looked at us before ordering us to change into bikinis. No questions. No ID. He didn't need to. With just a glance he had decided I was good enough. It became very clear to me, my worth wasn't about who I was, or what I could do, it was wrapped up in how I looked. That was all that mattered, and it was enough for him to let me work in his bar, confirming my appearance was my greatest asset, the only thing of value I had to offer.

The moment I stepped onto that stage, the men, most of them much older, turned their eyes toward me. For the first time in my life, I felt truly seen, like I had power. Their gaze was heavy, and for a girl who had always craved attention, it felt intoxicating. I could feel their desire, their admiration, and for a fleeting moment, I was the center of their world. I was someone who mattered. The validation from these older men, men who exuded experience and confidence, filled a void in me that I hadn't even realized was so deep.

When we first arrived, they told us we needed stage names, something exotic, something mysterious. It felt surreal, like stepping into a role I didn't yet understand. I was already struggling to figure out who I was, who Erin was, outside of the identity I had shared with my sister for so long. Suddenly, I had to invent someone new. It was thrilling and terrifying at the same time. The persona I created became a mask I wore, hiding the insecurity and uncertainty I felt beneath it.

On that stage, I wasn't just a girl anymore. I was a fantasy, a projection of what they wanted. I gave them a name, a story, a life I had made up on the spot, and in return, they gave me their attention, their admiration. I learned quickly what each man wanted to hear, how to make them feel special, desired. It was a game, a dangerous, seductive game and I adapted fast. But with every night that passed, I could feel myself slipping further away from the real me. In their eyes, I could be anyone, anything they needed. Yet, with every gaze, with every story I spun, I was slowly losing sight of who I truly was.

How could one decision, one fleeting moment, dictate how I would feel about myself for the next thirty years? His blue eyes, my dad's blue eyes, locking onto mine like a spotlight. They were the same eyes that had watched over me as a child, the same piercing gaze that always seemed to see right through me. But in that moment, they weren't protective or reassuring. They were filled with disappointment, and it felt like those eyes had never been colder. His voice followed, steady but sharp, burning me with shame.

The shock of seeing him standing there, my dad, of all people, stopped me cold. I felt paralyzed, that's how intense the shame was. My mind raced. How long had he been there? What had he seen? Every question hit me all at once, crashing into each other. I was caught, and there was no way out.

After slipping out of the bar unseen, we arrived at my boyfriend's house. But the fear hadn't left me. It gripped me tightly, refusing to let go. My dad didn't know exactly where my boyfriend lived, but he knew the town, and that was enough to keep me on edge. I've never been so scared. I couldn't shake the feeling that he was out there, searching for me, waiting to confront me again. I hardly slept that night, my mind replaying the scene over and over, knowing that in a moment, my life had changed forever.

The car I was driving, the one my dad had given me, felt like a ticking time bomb. Every moment I kept it, I was sure he'd report it stolen or demand it back. It wasn't just a car anymore. It was a symbol of everything that had just come crashing down, and there was no way to undo it.

At the moment I saw his eyes, I knew I couldn't live at home anymore. My dad had always told me, "You can be anything, but don't be a liar. I hate liars." And I had lied, over and over. I knew he would never forgive me for that. The trust between us was shattered, and with it, any sense of freedom I had left. I could already feel the walls closing in. My ability to come and go as I pleased would be gone and every move I made would be watched. The taste of freedom I had just experienced while dancing would be a distant memory. I had no choice. Living at home was no longer an option, I had to move out.

The next morning, I had to face the music. I called home, knowing I couldn't avoid it any longer. When my dad picked up the phone, I said,

"Hi," but he didn't respond. For a moment, I thought he'd hung up. Then my mom got on the line. Her voice, so familiar and usually so comforting but this time it sounded different to me—distant, concerned, hurt. I told her I was coming home to bring the car back and that I was moving out. She told me I didn't have to but I knew different. I didn't feel disowned or cast aside but I knew I had broken the trust, and if I stayed, I'd be trapped under my dad's strict rules forever. I couldn't imagine how I would ever gain his trust back or if he would even let me. I didn't see any other option but to leave and start living my life on my own.

Later that day, I brought the car home and packed up my things. My mom cried, my sister cried, but my dad... He barely looked at me. The feelings of disappointment and disapproval hung in the air, thick and suffocating. The only words he said to me that night were, "If you ever go back to one of those bars, I'll drag you out myself."

Those words stuck with me for years. They echoed in my mind every time I thought about that night. They were the only ones he ever spoke about that night, the only time he ever acknowledged what happened. After that we never talked about it again. I carried the shame and judgment with me, suffocating my sense of self for years. I lived as that seventeen year old girl for most of my life, unable to escape the weight of his gaze.

Not only did I leave my parents that night, I left my sister, the person who had been by my side from the moment she was born. Leaving her behind was harder than I realized. I left her to face the rumors and gossip that followed my decision to drop out of high school and move away. What I didn't understand at the time was the sense of abandonment she must have felt when I left. In an instant, she was without me for the first time in her life. She had to defend me while dealing with the judgment of others, all while coping with being alone. It's something I never fully considered back then, and only later in life did I truly begin to understand the weight of what she went through, further feeding my shame.

From that day forward, my relationship with my dad became strained. It took months before he would truly speak to me again. The unspoken tension was always there, hovering like a weight neither of us acknowledged. To this day, we've never talked about what happened that night.

I met my now ex-husband shortly after that, through the boyfriend who helped me escape that night. He was a musician, and I was an aspiring model. We chased our dreams all the way to Los Angeles, where we lived for three years. Living there was thrilling, there was an energy in the air that made everything seem possible. The city felt like it was pulsing with opportunity and for a while, I truly believed we could build a life there. I loved the pace—calm, yet with constant movement, and the way everything glittered with the sense of possibility. There was always this sense of something bigger just within reach. I felt a sense of adventure from the second we arrived and I fell in love with the idea that success could be just around the corner. For a while I felt like I could carve out a future in this place that seemed to hold the key to all my dreams coming true. But eventually, it became clear that the stability I craved and the family I wanted to eventually have would only really be possible in Canada. We needed to return home.

We moved back to Canada, and after some time had passed and the yearning of returning to Los Angeles had dissipated we had two beautiful boys. Life shifted dramatically. Being married to a "rockstar" was fun in my teens and twenties, but once the boys were born, I wanted something more—stability, a real family life. His lifestyle of late nights, coming home at four a.m., and the uncertainty of his income didn't match the life I envisioned for our boys and our family. I found myself working multiple jobs to help keep the family afloat, which wasn't what I ever wanted. Eventually, it became clear that we were on different paths, and we parted ways.

A few short months after my ex-husband moved out, my world was shattered. I was teaching a fitness class when my sister called, her voice breaking as she told me our mom had died. I couldn't process it. *Our Mom had died*, I thought, trying to process this unspeakable notion. *No she wasn't dead, she was safe in a nursing home being looked after.* Rationalizing this horror, I tried to make sense of what I'd just heard, but the more I battled with it, the more intense the feeling became. It was as if my mind and body were at war. The logical part of me attempted to process the news, while my entire nervous system screamed in despair. All I could think at the time was that I had to finish teaching this class; I couldn't let down these ladies or my boss. So, that's what I did. I pushed it all down and taught as if nothing had happened. Looking back now, this was one instant that stood out where I abandoned myself, without giving any concern or consideration to what I needed at that time. My people-pleasing and fear of disappointing someone had become a significant part of who I was by this time in my life and this experience was evidence of that.

Afterward, I spoke to my dad who couldn't bear the thought of going to the nursing home to release her body. "I've seen enough dead bodies in my career and I don't want to see hers," he said. So, I went in his place. I didn't have a choice. He did not protect me from what I was about to see, knowing the horrific impact it would have on me. The image of her lying in that bed is something I will never forget. It's burned into my mind as my last memory of her.

I didn't have the space to truly grieve or process her death. I had just recently separated from my husband two months prior and had two little boys to take care of and was struggling to keep things afloat. I pushed my grief aside, not realizing how deeply that decision would affect me.

After a few months of working and struggling, I knew I needed stability for myself and my boys. That's when I decided to become a police officer. I worked incredibly hard to get that job, all while navigating a nasty divorce and custody battle with my ex. But when I finally earned the badge, it felt like a huge accomplishment.

Throughout my life, my appearance had always been the first thing people noticed about me. Compliments on my looks were constant, and I began to feel that my value was tied solely to how I presented myself. This set the stage for an innate belief I had about myself that my worth was tied up in how I looked. Even my dad, watching me play basketball, would say things like, "Well, the shot looked good, too bad it didn't go in." It was as if my efforts and skills were overshadowed by how I looked doing them. This constant emphasis on appearance made me believe that beauty was my only asset.

Becoming a police officer changed that narrative for me. I identified so deeply with the role of helping others. For the first time I felt like people took me seriously, not because of how I looked, but because of what I was capable of. I had earned my worth through determination and hard work. I had finally become something more than my appearance.

Those early years on the job were tough. My first posting was in the Northwest Region, about four hours northeast of Thunder Bay, Ontario. I didn't know anyone, I had no family or friends there, but in small communities like that, police officers are often embraced by locals and the policing community itself supported each other. Thankfully, I found a young girl in town to help take care of my boys while I was working. Still, being a single mom made things challenging.

As a new officer I felt the weight of needing to prove myself. Those early years are difficult for everyone but for me it felt especially intense. At thirty-seven, I was older than most rookies. I was a woman, a single mom, and I felt like I had so much more to prove. I had to show that I was worthy of the job, that I deserved to be there.

In reality I was capable and qualified, but my past, the shame I still carried from that seventeen year old girl who worked as an exotic dancer made me feel like I had to work that much harder. I thought if I just excelled, if I pushed myself harder, maybe I could finally shed that old identity that I carried. Becoming a police officer felt like my first real chance to be taken seriously. It certainly didn't help that when my ex-husband found out I was trying to get hired, he laughed and said no one would take me seriously. It was something I believed people would be proud of, a real accomplishment. Finally, I thought people would look at me and say that I'd actually done something with my life.

But in striving so hard to prove my worth, I started to tie my identity to the job. Being a police officer became more than just a career, it became my validation. The role reinforced the belief that my value was wrapped up in what I did, not who I was. Just as I had once relied on my appearance to attract attention and approval, I now depended on my professional accomplishments to feel worthy. With every success feeding the notion that I was only as good as my latest achievement; I threw myself into work with the same passion I once applied to perfecting my image, still seeking external validation and molding myself to fit what I thought the world wanted me to be. Deep down, I hadn't addressed the core issues, the lingering belief that who I was at my essence wasn't enough. Whether through looks or achievement, I was continually looking for external validation for my self-worth, repeating the same patterns in a different setting.

The shame I carried from that night in the bar forced me to create someone other than who I really was, because that girl, the girl I had been, when I was doing what I wanted, what felt authentic to me at that time, was someone we didn't talk about. That girl was shameful. So, when I was hired as a police officer, my perfectionism and people-pleasing tendencies made me the ideal candidate. I always said yes, never no. I overworked, over-achieved, driven by an intense need to prove I wasn't that seventeen year old girl from the bar. I wasn't her anymore. I couldn't be. But even as I tried to bury that part of me, the shame lingered, pushing me to excel at everything.

I knew there were officers in my service who had been in high school with me when I left, who had heard the rumors about why I had disappeared. Even though I was working in a detachment far from my hometown, the interconnected nature of our police service meant that distance offered little protection. We frequently attended courses and training sessions where officers from all over the province gathered. It wasn't uncommon to find myself sitting next to someone from my hometown detachment. In those settings, casual conversations could easily drift into sharing stories and gossip. I feared that my name might come up, that someone might mention the girl who left under mysterious circumstances, sparking curiosity or recognition.

The thought of being the topic of discussion among colleagues sent a cold shiver down my spine. Why wouldn't someone say something when they found out I had become a police officer? My fear was so strong that it bordered on paranoia, but it was real to me. I lived with the constant worry that my past would be unearthed, that whispers would spread like wildfire through the ranks. Our service was vast, but news, especially the gossip-kind, had a way of traveling quickly.

This fear was ignited early in my career, during my time at police college. My relationship with my ex-husband was strained. We had finished a messy custody battle, where I was awarded sole custody but while I was training he had the boys during the week. One weekend, when I went to pick them up, he stopped me with a cruel smile and said, "What do you think the police would say if they found out you didn't disclose your job as an exotic dancer?" His words hit me like a punch to the gut. Instantly, I was transported back to that night when my dad had caught me—the shame, the terror. I had worked so hard to build a stable life for our boys, and now it felt like everything could be ripped away. Could he really do this? Would he try to destroy everything I'd built, just because he was angry?

That moment with my ex-husband brought my deepest fears to the forefront, shaking any sense of security I might have had. From the very start of my policing career, I was reminded of the secret I was desperately trying to keep hidden. It caused me to become hyper aware of the possibilities, my footing unsteady as I navigated this new world. The fear wasn't just a distant worry, it was a constant companion, prompted by his threat and realizing that people I knew before were now my coworkers.

At work, when my platoon mates casually chatted about exotic dancers or joked about bars like the one I'd worked in, I'd freeze. Do they know?

Are they testing me? Watching how I react? The paranoia was intense, but I couldn't shake the feeling that I was under scrutiny, that any slip-up could expose me. I lived in a perpetual state of hypervigilance, always anticipating the moment someone would say, "I know."

For years, the weight of that threat loomed over me, amplifying the shame I already carried. It pushed me to work harder, to be better, in the desperate hope that if anyone ever heard those rumors, they wouldn't believe them. My perfectionism and people-pleasing tendencies thrived in the police world. The harder I worked, the more recognition I received, which only compelled me to push myself further. I overachieved, not out of passion, but out of a frantic need for validation and an effort to outrun my past. I thought that if my work spoke for itself, then my history wouldn't matter. Yet, the fear of being discovered never left me. It lingered, a shadow following me every time I put on my uniform. And it worked, until it didn't.

I'll never forget the day my body finally gave up on me. For years, the signs had been there, subtle, quiet warnings I didn't fully understand. I remember one evening vividly, my now-husband and I were out for a run. He had just recovered from knee surgery a few months prior and was getting back into his routine, but I was the one struggling. My legs felt heavy, like they were weighed down with lead, and he had to help me up the hills. I couldn't wrap my head around it. Running had always been my thing. I was a marathon runner.I ran in the Police Memorial Run every year. But suddenly, I couldn't do it. Slowly, my body started giving me more signs. I felt sick at the thought of going to work, headaches would creep in, my hair was falling out. Looking back, my body had been begging me to slow down, trying to warn me that the overdrive of overcompensating I was living in couldn't last forever. And then, came the day when my body finally said, enough.

I'll never forget the day everything finally shut down. For years, I had poured my heart and soul into my work, driven by a growing passion for traffic safety. Traffic had become more than just a part of my job, it was my calling. I immersed myself in specialized training, led provincial initiatives, and consistently exceeded expectations in traffic enforcement. My dedication didn't go unnoticed. I was recognized for my achievements and, eventually, offered a Temporary Acting Assignment (TAA) in the dedicated Traffic Unit.

This TAA was my dream job; the position I had always aspired to. It was the culmination of all my hard work and the stepping stone toward a permanent role in the unit. Accepting the TAA felt like everything was finally falling into place. I was being groomed for the specialty I was so passionate about, and I was determined to prove that I was worthy of the position.

However, along with the TAA came new pressures I hadn't fully anticipated. I was being pushed to specialize in collision reconstruction, a highly technical field requiring advanced mathematical skills. Deep down, I didn't think I was ready. I lacked the years of experience in collision investigations that I believed were necessary. Math had never been my strong suit, and the thought of diving into such complex work was daunting.

I tried to voice my concerns, telling my superiors that I didn't feel prepared for this specialty. But my people-pleasing nature and fear of jeopardizing my dream job kept me from pushing back too hard. I sensed that agreeing to take on reconstruction was expected of me, that it was the only way to secure my place in the unit. Despite my reservations, I agreed, knowing full well that this type of work didn't come easy to me.

I had to work twice as hard to grasp the concepts, spending countless hours studying and practicing. While I loved every other aspect of traffic and enforcement, reconstruction was a constant struggle. It was made clear to me that I didn't have a choice if I wanted to continue pursuing my dream in the Traffic Unit. I sacrificed everything, my personal life, my family, my sleep, my health, to excel in this role. I overachieved at every turn, driven by an endless need for validation.

In the months leading up to that day, my sergeant and I had countless talks about the pressure I was under, how overwhelmed I felt, and how the stress was mounting. Those conversations often ended with me in tears, feeling more like she doubted my capabilities than was concerned for my well-being. That only made me push myself harder.

Then came the day when everything unraveled. My sergeant asked to speak with me, and we went car-to-car, lining up our driver's windows so we could talk privately—something we always did when we needed discretion at work. I felt sick to my stomach. This conversation felt different. "We need to talk about your TAA," she began, her tone unreadable. She told me that upper management had decided I wasn't performing my temporary assignment correctly, a claim that was a complete and utter lie. The TAA I had worked so hard for, the one they'd promised would be mine until a permanent spot became available, was over. Just like that.

The rug was pulled out from under me in one sentence. I sat there, stunned. I had given everything for that position, for that unit, for the specialty I was so passionate about. And now, through a car window, I was being told that none of it mattered. There was no meeting, no discussion, no formality. The decision had been made, and that was final. I felt like a pawn in a game I knew nothing about.

After years of jumping through hoops and proving myself, the betrayal by management was the final blow. Despite all my efforts, I no longer fit into their agenda anymore. I was disposed of. When my sergeant uttered the words, "The TAA is over," my body gave out. I can't even remember what I said or did next, except that I knew I had to leave. I needed to go home. At that moment, my body completely shut down. It no longer felt like mine. I had a total breakdown, a moment where I realized that everything I had been pushing myself through for all those years had finally caught up to me, and my body simply couldn't take it anymore. If I am being honest, the last thirty-four years had finally caught up to me.

I was forty-four years old when this happened and the stress I carried finally overwhelmed me. It all started when I was ten years old, the year my mother was diagnosed with multiple sclerosis. At that tender age, I began to learn that to be noticed, to be accepted, to be loved, I had to please others. My mother's illness consumed so much of our family's attention that I felt invisible unless I did something exceptional. This people-pleasing nature was further fueled by that pivotal moment when my father caught me dancing at that bar. The shame from that night deepened my belief that I wasn't good enough, reinforcing my need to mold myself to meet others expectations.

Over the next thirty-four years, I perfected the art of being what others wanted me to be. I molded myself to fit expectations, first to gain my family's attention, then to earn approval from peers, teachers, partners, and eventually, my superiors at work. My entire life had been a relentless pursuit of acceptance, driven by a deep-seated belief that I wasn't enough as I was. Whether it was through my appearance or my professional achievements, I sought validation from the outside world, always trying to be someone else to gain love and respect.

So when my body gave out that day, it wasn't just the immediate stress or the betrayal by management, it was the cumulative effect of a lifetime spent neglecting my own needs and authenticity. The girl who learned to people-please, to cope with her mother's illness, and to hide her shame from that night with my dad had grown into a woman who didn't know how to stop. And at forty-four, the facade could no longer hold. The years of suppressing my true self, of constantly overcompensating, had finally taken its toll.

Looking back now, I realize that if I had been a healthy officer, someone who set boundaries, took care of myself, and knew how to manage stress, I likely could have handled that situation differently. But I wasn't. My life as a police officer had become like a game of Jenga. Each traumatic incident, each moment of intense stress, was like pulling out another piece of the tower. You never know which piece will make everything collapse, but eventually, one will. And that's exactly what happened that day. It wasn't the biggest, most obvious moment that brought me down, it was the one I didn't see coming, the one that caused everything to fall apart.

Going on leave signaled the end of my relentless efforts and the start of an overwhelming crisis. After that devastating conversation with my sergeant, I rushed to see my doctor, terrified of what was happening to me. I left work in tears, hardly recognizing the person I had become. My doctor barely recognized me too, not just because I was physically exhausted, but because my spirit was shattered. I was placed on sick leave to deal with severe burnout and emotional turmoil. I would later be diagnosed with Post Traumatic Stress Disorder, anxiety, and depression. This sudden time away from work was the first clear sign that years of people-pleasing and wearing masks had completely drained me. I wasn't sleeping, I was crying uncontrollably, and I spent my days in pajamas, binge-watching Netflix, and eating junk food. Without the job, I didn't know who I was anymore and I began to question if I ever really knew.

While I was off work, everything started falling apart. The police service showed little support, stripping away everything that made me feel like I had any worth. Letters and calls from management asking for my gear, laptop, and even random equipment came relentlessly. It felt like I was being erased, one piece at a time.

In the midst of all this, my sister told me she had made the difficult decision to pursue Medical Assistance in Dying (MAiD), a legal process that allows individuals with severe, incurable illnesses to choose to end their lives with medical support. Although I wasn't entirely familiar with MAiD myself, I understood that she was seeking control over her suffering and hoping to find peace on her own terms. When she was in her early twenties she too was diagnosed with MS, but at the time we all had so much hope that things would be different for her than they were for our mom. She fought the disease with all she had. Read all the newest research and traveled to a few countries for radical treatments but in the end, she too became debilitated, unable to walk, finally bound to a wheelchair. The difference between her and our mom was that she knew how much worse it would get, she watched our mom deteriorate and ultimately need twenty-four hour care. My sister always said she would never end up in a nursing home. I begged her to reconsider, to think about her daughter and all of us who loved her. I became desperate, telling her I would move in with her, move closer, anything to be there for her more. But with the calmest voice and unwavering assurance she said, "No, I can't live like this anymore, I'm in pain every day and every day feels the same. This isn't living, it's existing."

I begged her to reconsider, telling her how much her daughter needed her, how she needed to see her graduate high school, at least. But she replied, "Erin, there will always be another milestone, something else that keeps me here. But the truth is there will never be a perfect time and it's only going to get worse." So, with dignity and grace, on October 22, 2020, the anniversary of our mom's death, my sister ended her battle with MS, on her own terms.

Grief entered my life like a tidal wave, and I was unprepared for the force of it. I found myself grieving the loss of my sister and my mother at the same time. It was like everything came crashing down all at once, my family, my job, my sense of self. I had already been diagnosed with PTSD, but most days, I didn't know what I was grieving more, the loss of my sister, my mother, my career, or the complex trauma from years of police work. The horrific scenes I had witnessed as an officer piled onto the other traumas, and the weight was unbearable.

Those next few years were some of the darkest of my life, but they also became a turning point. I was determined not to let the pain consume me. Instead, I cracked myself open, surrendered, and began to see clearly for the first time how I had played a role in my own burnout. I sought out therapy—talk therapy, group therapy, and even alternative methods like ayahuasca and ketamine therapy. I practiced yoga, meditation, and focused on nutrition. I tried everything because my police service offered me no support or assistance during this incredibly lonely time. Left to navigate my struggles alone, I felt deeply embarrassed and like a failure, without any help from the very organization I had dedicated so much of my life to.

Through therapy, I began to realize how I had allowed things to unfold, not just at work, but throughout my entire life. I could see that I was never truly my authentic self. I wore a mask, always trying to be the good girl, the person people would approve of and respect. All of this was driven by the shame I carried and how I still identified with that seventeen year old girl who was caught in that bar.

Living an inauthentic life led me to places where anger, fear, shame, and guilt all collided, and eventually, it brought me to my knees. I'm grateful, in a strange way, that the police service became the runaway train that derailed me, because it forced me to confront the truth: I wasn't living for myself. I was living to gain love, respect, and validation, all based on a false version of myself.

It took immense courage and vulnerability to admit that I had been hiding behind masks for most of my life. The energy it took to maintain those masks was exhausting, and it nearly killed me. But with time, therapy, and introspection, I began to peel back the layers and finally understand who I truly am. It has been a painful process, but it has also been liberating. For the first time, I accepted that I have every right to feel the way I do. My childhood, the constant need to be noticed, the survival mode I lived in for most of my life, it all makes sense now.

I began to release the shame I had carried for over thirty years, the shame tied to that seventeen year old girl who had made a choice. I am no longer ashamed of it. That decision, while misunderstood by many, was my way of empowering myself. I now give myself grace and understanding, and I take time every day to ask myself if I am living authentically and if what I am doing is for myself or for someone else.

I wasn't put on this Earth to please people. I was put here to learn from my experiences and live as my true, authentic self. Dropping the masks and standing in my truth has been the most freeing journey of my life. The healing has been immense. The trauma will always be a part of me, and the tendency to slip into old patterns is still there. But now, I consciously tap into my own energy, my authentic self, and ask, "What do I want?"

In the end, I even thank the command staff at my service for making the decisions they did. Their choices, though painful at the time, ultimately freed me from a life I was no longer meant to live. They allowed me to break free from the chains of perfectionism, people-pleasing, and shame. And now, I stand in my truth, stronger, braver, and more authentic than ever before.

But through it all, I've come to realize that everything happens for a reason. I believe the universe brings us to where we need to be, even if the journey is painful. Losing my sister, dealing with PTSD, and all the other challenges I've faced have brought me to a place of gratitude. I feel my sister and mom's presence around me all the time, and I'm learning to honor myself in a way I never have before.

For years, I ran myself into the ground trying to please everyone else. Now, I'm learning to ask myself what I need, and that is enough. If I have the capacity to serve others, I will. But if I don't, that's okay too. I'm finally giving myself permission to be tired, to take breaks, to be human.

It's been a long journey, but I'm finally finding peace.

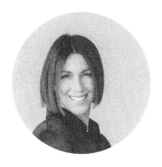

ERIN GORRIE

Erin is a police officer currently on medical leave due to a workplace injury. She is a dedicated mother of two wonderful young adults, and a certified 200-hour yoga instructor. Over the past four years, she has embarked on a transformative mental health journey, discovering the healing power of yoga and founding Muskoka Puppy Yoga, a unique initiative that combines yoga practice with the therapeutic companionship of puppies. Erin is passionate about supporting others, especially first responders, who she aims to help navigate their mental health journeys and foster environments where no one feels alone. Believing her experiences have guided her to where she is meant to be, she uses her story and work to inspire strength, joy, and authenticity in others. Connect with Erin at www.muskokapuppyyoga.ca or on Instagram @muskokapuppyyoga.

Presence lacks fear, and presence is love.

Sensitivity Advisory: This chapter references personal experiences of death of a parent and cancer.

CHAPTER SEVEN

Inhale Love, Exhale Gratitude

Written by Lesa Mueller

There's still a part of me that feels my blood boil when I think about the doctor that she saw for years and years. Why did he not pick up on the signs of her decline and dig deeper into the causes. He should have known her well enough to know this wasn't normal for her. She lived an active healthy lifestyle, a good cook, and ate well. Then the guilt sets in, I saw the decline also, and I did nothing; until it was too late. I should have pushed harder. I should have advocated more. I should have...

I could see that my mother was losing weight, she was becoming frail. Twelve years earlier she had successfully navigated breast cancer. She reassured us that she was doing the things she needed to do, having regular doctor visits, and a checkup with an all clear signal before heading south for the winter.

Sometimes in life we are handed something that feels so big, so heavy to carry, yet in the moment, somehow we find the strength to do what is needed. I also realize that the things that feel the hardest, the things that often infuriate us are the very things that push us into a greater sense of purpose, or direction. These feelings are what brought me to want to write this chapter. This experience was a deep reminder to me how important it is to advocate for those we love.

Even though I am so grateful for our medical system and all the ways that we have access to the things we need. There are so many good and beautiful things about those humans that provide our medical care, but they are still human. They don't have all the answers. Mistakes are made.

The reality is, that you know your body better than anyone. I see my parents' generation believing wholeheartedly in their doctors. That what they say is written in stone; that there is no need for questioning or second opinions, no need to push back or ask for more. I realize now how much this generation needs us, our voices, our strengths, our courage, our ability to know in our gut and trust it. We know ourselves and our people better than a doctor who is meeting us for a ten minute appointment ever could.

As my parents left for Arizona with that clean bill of health, I could feel that something wasn't right. I didn't want them to go. I could even feel there was hesitation from Mom, she wasn't as eager to go as in the past. Did she have a feeling that deep inside that there was more going on? I believe she did subconsciously. When I look back at her actions last fall, I believe she knew. I think I did too.

Mom had some health complications while in Arizona and spent a few days in hospital. Although the staff there said she was fine, within days she was experiencing the same terrible symptoms that landed her in hospital less than a week before. At the end of January 2024 my parents flew home from Arizona. I won't ever forget the fear in my Dad's voice that morning he called, within hours they were at the airport heading home. In the days to come Mom was diagnosed with stage four cancer, a diagnosis no one wants to hear. Again, strangely, I already knew in my heart... or my gut.

Mom was one of the most positive people I have ever known, she rarely let things ruffle her feathers. She seemed to be able to let things go and find peace, something I know she practiced with intention, but nonetheless she was able to do. She started treatment that would hopefully slow the cancer, give us more time. Initially she indicated that she felt like she had a couple years left on Earth with us. Was that her optimism or hope? I won't know now.

In the next few months we could see her steady decline. The women in the family had this inner knowing that her time remaining with us was going to be short. The men on the other hand, didn't appear to see it the same. Maybe they were holding strong to the hope that treatments would slow the cancer and we would have more time. It was a bold reminder of how we each see things and process differently. It was also a reminder to trust my intuition; to trust my gut.

As we walked this path, we could have been consumed by anger and frustration at the lack of diagnoses earlier, one that could have changed the trajectory of her life, but we chose to come from a place of acceptance of what is and where we were. Although I still reflect on what we could have done differently—knowing that had I stepped in sooner, maybe pushed a little harder, been respectfully bossy, and listened to my gut, maybe things would have been different. Maybe we could have had just a little more time. Knowing when to step in and step up is so tricky, especially with our elders. People who have raised us, taught us respect, guided us, been our role models. We want to offer privacy, yet the difficulty in not being part of doctor appointments and first-hand information was so hard. There is such a fine line about how we can step in respectfully.

When we hear something, we only take in a small percentage of what is being said. There's only so much we can process, then it is filtered through our own lenses of what we want to hear. How are we interpreting what we heard? Often we hear part of a conversation but we get hung up on one word or phrase that may send us into paralysis from hearing anything further. When we are in a state of stress, trauma, or grief it is difficult for us to have full access to our brain, we may be in fight, flight, or freeze. Now let's multiply that with other complications like age, illness symptoms, and terminology. Are we able to ask the right questions and hear the answers with understanding and clarity?

It's easy to think we can do things on our own, because we can, but that doesn't mean we should. Some people don't want to burden others, some people are private, but when it comes down to receiving information will you be able to accurately share that information afterward with those who also need the information? I wish I had been at more doctors appointments to help listen, translate, and offer suggestions. I wish I had been a stronger advocate; it might be one of the best gifts we could give our loved ones. I remember in several appointments over the years with various family members I heard the doctor ask, "What would you like us to do?" I remember family members not knowing how to respond, and that by me being there allowed us to ask questions that helped create clarity so that a plan could be made. It's not anyone's fault; we expect the doctors to have all the answers. There is no magic in medicine, sometimes it is merely trial and error when it comes to determining a diagnosis and the next steps. Sometimes we need to provide input and advocate for the best options. Sometimes we need to push a little to make certain things happen. Sometimes we need to be able to follow up. This is the current reality of our healthcare system. If you aren't at those appointments you miss the opportunity to do these things, you miss the first-hand information and the input into the care of your loved ones.

In the last stages of Mom's journey I remember feeling like her doctor wasn't doing enough and questioning why certain things weren't happening. I had been trusting what was being shared with us until it just didn't make sense any longer. I knew my Mom's wishes were not to prolong her suffering. What time she had left, she wanted to be about quality of life, and I could respect that. I also knew it didn't have to be this hard. It wasn't until then that I really saw how she and Dad had taken on so much of this journey privately, so much more than any of us even knew. My Dad had been amazing in how he supported Mom. I wish I had known sooner as we could have taken so much of the burden off them. She could have been more comfortable. It didn't need to be this hard. So there it is, that fine line of allowing them their privacy, or pushing our way in a little more.

Not everyone gets the opportunity to say goodbye. Many people are gone before we even know it's on the horizon. Not everyone gets to surround themselves with those they love and share stories, memories, and say what's on their heart. We truly made the most of Mom's last few weeks for which I will be eternally grateful. My sister and I each got to curl her hair for the first time and help her feel as beautiful as she truly was. We talked about who she was most looking forward to seeing in heaven and what we were most grateful for. I got to hold her hand as she took her last breath and she knew how loved she truly was. Inhale love, exhale gratitude.

Like she had each day of our lives, she had everything in place. She made things easy for us, her selfless acts, and preparation. The signs were there months before that she was preparing, but I didn't see them at first. She wrote us all letters that we will cherish until our last breath. She asked when I was wrapping up certain projects, and back from this or that, when my brother would be finished seeding the crops. She was looking for her window. Her window when we would all be okay to say goodbye. I believe in her last months she knew deep down when her time would come. She was clear. She was at peace. Even the day we carried her out of the house, knowing it would be her last time in the home she raised us. The home she gathered her loved ones in. The home where so many memories were made, so many meals shared, and moments lived. She was still smiling the day we left home until the moment she left us forever.

With a deep breath, I could come back to presence, and be in the moment because presence lacks fear, and presence is love. The care our family provided in her last weeks made her final journey the best it could possibly be. Only those truly close to her would know the little things that would bring her comfort. While I know that not everyone could do the things we did, we are wired to do hard things. Being there for those we love is the best gift we can ever provide. Those that have spent a lifetime loving us, the least we can do is give them our presence, our time, our love in their darkest hour.

As a caregiver, I feel like my grief was delayed. I was so focused on Mom and Dad and orchestrating all the things, that there wasn't space for grief in the time of her care and transition. I still need to remind myself to be kind to myself and honor the time and space that I need. We all grieve differently and at different paces. Most importantly, I can now recognize and honor each person's journey through grief. No two people will have the same experience, and that we each do the best we can each day. I practice inhaling love and exhaling gratitude each day, and check on my people regularly. Although some of my family members don't share much, we still need each other, just maybe differently. Going silent for long periods however, is not good for anyone. My journey as a certified coach has taught me how valuable the spoken word is. When we speak the words they land in our body and mind differently than if we just think them. It helps us process, understand, and move forward in ways we might not otherwise be able to. As I reflect back on those who have checked in on me, I am so grateful that they took the time to ask what I needed from them. I'm eternally grateful for everyone who attended Mom's celebration of life, sent cards, and made donations in her memory; these gestures meant so much to us.

You often hear people say they don't want a memorial or funeral held for them when they pass away. These services are not for the departed, they are for those left behind. Those filled with grief and a longing to keep memories alive. In my community it was common practice to hold a service within about a week following death, once details were in order. Through the pandemic, it became common for many to put a service on hold in hopes that in time people could truly celebrate their loved one with as many people as possible when we were able to gather again in large groups. I believe that this made room for changing the expectation of what *should be* to what *feels best* for individual situations. Our family wasn't ready to rush the process of having a service when we lost Mom; her wish to be cremated allowed us time to pause. It gave us time to grieve and spend time planning a celebration that truly reflected her life. I don't think we would have achieved this to the level we did if we had a service right away. There was too much grief, our thoughts were scattered. Waiting allowed us to truly focus on the beautiful woman that she truly was. This reminded me that it's okay to pause and take the time that we need in life and in death.

Daily I still reach for the phone to call her, and I think of her countless times throughout each day. Some days, memories come falling from my eyes unexpectedly at the grocery store, or event that I'm at. When my heart aches to hug her I lean into gratitude to be thankful for the time we had, the impact she made in so many lives, and know that I'm not the only one missing her. I lean into all that she taught me, the memories, and her zest for life, and it reminds me to live out loud each day. She was the inspiration for my previous chapter titled, Live Out Loud, in volume one of this book series.

Mom not only taught us how to live, she also taught us how to die. It was a reflection of her life; she lived each moment until her last breath with such grace, such gratitude, and so much love. Being able to honor the wishes of our loved ones and helping them through those difficult times is the most humbling gift we could give. Walking my Mom home was truly the most difficult, and most beautiful gift she gave me. It was such an honor to be able to love on her how she always loved on me.

If you are navigating a relationship with a loved one who is walking the path of a diagnosis, if you are caring for an aging parent, or if you are walking someone home, know that you are not alone. Remember to follow and trust your gut instinct and that you know your people better than anyone else. Keep communicating and step in when you know the time is right, and have the courage to do so. Always be respectful, but it's okay to be firm; remember how you will want to be treated when it's your turn to go down this path. Be open to seeing things from their perspective and honor their wishes as best you can. Help them seek clarity and gain other perspectives. Know that you can do the hard things when you need to, even if you think you can't possibly. Allow yourself to grieve. It is a process and each person will be on their own path. There is no right way to do this, other than be kind to yourself and others. We all do the best that we can. Know that in the weeks, days, and months to come your people will need you. Find moments of gratitude along the way, that is where the beauty is. And finally, be present in the moment, before the moments are gone and they are no longer here with you. Peace and love my friends.

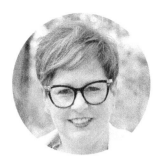

LESA MUELLER

Lesa grew up outside of a small town in rural Alberta where she learned to love gardening, nature, and animals. Lesa is a recovering perfectionist, and she finds joy in creating safe spaces, exploring ideas and opportunities, and collaborating with others. This stands true in all aspects of her life as she wears many hats. Lesa is the CEO and a Certified Travel Counsellor with Stonegate Tours along with owner of Lesa Mueller Consulting and Coaching where she's a Certified Leadership Coach, mentor, facilitator, and consultant. She's also a wife, mother and ecstatic to be a grandmother to five grandsons. You can connect with Lesa at www.lesamueller.com, www.live-outloud.com, and www.stonegatetours.com.

Photo credit: Pretty as a Picture Photography

I kept putting off living my life until I had the perfect life and the perfect body. Guess what? Perfect never came.

CHAPTER EIGHT

Beyond the Looking Glass: Loving Yourself from the Inside Out

Written by Laura Tolosi

I can picture myself at seven years old sitting in the bathroom, looking at my mom as she meticulously put her makeup on. I loved watching her. I thought she was the most beautiful mom in the world and I couldn't wait to grow up and put makeup on like her.

Of course as many little girls do, we got into our moms eyeshadows and blushes, and played dress-up, wore her clothes, her lipstick, and, of course, her high heels. My sister and I often took out our mom's wedding gown and an old bridesmaid dress of hers and would walk around and pretend we were in the Miss America pageant. What fun we had masquerading around and pretending to be the belle of the ball. How fun it was to just be ourselves without a care, dressing up to emulate our beautiful mom, playing in our imaginary worlds, and having the very best times doing it.

Until one day the wind was taken from my innocent young girl's sail. I was playing with some friends on the block, and I was called a "blimp." The fun and games and innocence vanished, only to be replaced with guilt and shame and the beginning of years of hiding my body and sneaking food in the kitchen late at night when I thought everyone was sleeping. From that day on, I wore a gray zipped up sweatshirt at all times and always had a T-shirt over my bathing suit. In high school I felt so much jealousy of my other friends who could wear a bikini to the beach. Meanwhile there I was wearing a one-piece swimsuit, covered up with T-shirts, trying everything I could to blend in with the sand. I began Weight Watchers for the first time—I would eventually start it at least another three times by age sixteen, with my mom right alongside me. I'm not sure if she brought me for her

105

own unhappiness with herself, or to support me. It didn't matter, nothing stopped the guilt, shame, and embarrassment after a weekly weigh in where I didn't "make weight." To this day I make it a point to not do weekly weigh-ins and not to put any significance to that one measly number staring back at me.

On the outside I am sure I seemed like your typical, happy young girl. I did well in school. I had a lot of friends. And I did have fun. However, no one saw how I felt so much less-than because of my body shape. And no one saw how I turned to my true best friend, food, to soothe me and my emotions. When I didn't get asked to the prom one year by the boy I had secretly crushed on, or when the embarrassment and shame came over me when the dance instructor I admired addressed the entire class to say we needed to lose weight before our recital—knowing full well it was me she was referring to, I would turn to food as a way to make myself feel better.

Coming from an Italian American family didn't make it easy to even attempt to stay away from food. We loved food. My mom and grandmother were the best Italian cooks. I was blessed. I enjoyed my macaroni and meatballs a lot. I pretty much grew up on Cheese Doodles, ice cream, and soda. Food was around for good times, and food was always around for bad times. I had this love/hate relationship with it. I really loved eating my mom's and grandma's food, and my love to learn how to cook began with them, too. Yet, I felt like food was also the enemy. I couldn't stop eating when I was told to stop or when I thought I shouldn't eat, and the vicious emotional cycle of eating to soothe my soul continued. For years.

Enter college. And things began to change.

I was still enjoying food. I worked at KFC for extra cash and would bring home the leftover biscuits and extra crispy chicken any night I could. But I also began to run too. And I loved it. It was freeing and enjoyable and produced the endorphins that were much needed and missed. In high school I was dancing and playing sports, and had my endorphins attended too, however that was lost in the transition to college. Until I found running. The running began to change my body shape and my outlook on how I felt about myself; miraculous as it was when I look back now.

Add to that, my course of study in college? Biology.

I wanted to be a doctor. I wanted to help people with their health. And because I did truly love food, I took my first nutrition class. It was the hardest, yet best class I had ever taken, and lit a passion in me that I still have to this day. I finally saw the power to use our food as our medicine, not as our nemesis like many of us, especially women or people who struggle with overeating, are made to believe. I learned how food was used as a way to heal our bodies. And so on my own journey I began to use food to heal myself, to lose weight, and eventually change the trajectory of my life. I went from feeling inadequate to feeling excited, from making choices that finally felt good to my body and my mind, and it then reflected in my physical appearance as well. What a blessing it was enrolling in "Diet Therapy" with a professor who lit this fire inside me, in hindsight. I let go of becoming a doctor, and went full steam ahead into nutrition. I never looked back.

Food, plus physical activity? At that time, it was my home run.

I had always been an active kid. Playing sports, dancing, just running around. When I grew up, being active was just what we did. It's how we played. We ran around. Played hide-and-seek. Played cops and robbers with our bikes. We were always up to some activity or game. Always moving. Always running around. Playing was fun. Playing was active. Playing was outside in the summer all day long, and in the winter, as long as we could be out there without getting frost bitten. We loved to play. Exercise was not used as a way to try to manipulate our physical appearance, it was just what we did.

I had always loved moving my body, whether through play as a young child, organized sports and dance in high school, and running in college and after. When I realized moving my body was a source of fun that was missing in my life, I made it a priority again. As soon as my daughters were old enough for the day care at the gym, I got back into a routine of going regularly. I was with an amazing group of women, one more gorgeous than the other, all with strong, powerful bodies. They inspired me and made going to the gym even more fun for me.

One day we were all standing around chatting and I was listening to all these beautiful, strong, powerful women talking negatively about themselves in front of our very vulnerable toddler daughters. I felt like that little girl watching my mom put on her makeup and thinking she was the most beautiful woman in the world. And here I was with these amazing women thinking the very same thing about them, but they didn't see it. My heart sank because it hit me then. Our society has defined what beauty should look like and how we as moms subconsciously bought into this one-size-fits-all picture of beauty. Through our own negative self-talk, we have continued this incredibly vicious cycle of thinking that we don't measure up, that we are less-than, or not good enough. When really, we do and we are, and everyone around us sees it, but we often don't.

I finally saw how as women we came to think that our value, our worth, our love, is connected to how we physically look on the outside and just how much we hold in our feelings when we don't think we measure up. I was not excluded from this thinking. I was guilty of it too. It brought to the surface the memories of how I felt when I was called a blimp *and believed it about myself* and how many years it took me to come to terms with how my body was shaped and how to feel good in my body no matter the number on the scale. As I stood there listening to them, I was reminded of all those self-esteem crushing years and the subsequent feelings of shame and guilt, and the countless bites of food I used to soothe the emotions I didn't understand and pushed down because I had no way to process them and let them go. But as I listened to this conversation, I told myself that it had to stop, and it had to stop with me first.

I looked at my two innocent young daughters and knew it was time to heal these generational wounds around our body. I wanted my daughters, myself, and all women to be able to stand in front of that mirror and see the true beauty, not the beauty standards we've been told by society to aspire to. I wanted my daughters to love themselves wholly and completely just as they are. I wanted them to look beyond the skin that holds our bones in place and see to the heart because the heart is where the beauty really comes from. I wanted that for them, for the moms, and I also wanted that for me.

It's a very interesting cycle if you look at it; one much like the chicken or the egg— which came first? You see, we are bombarded in our society with these outside ideals of what beauty looks like, and then we look in the mirror, and don't measure up. We scrutinize every single thing. And we feel bad. We feel ashamed. We feel less-than. Unless we have a way to let go of these self loathing feelings, we look for ways to soothe ourselves. Hello Haagen Daz or Ben & Jerry's, take your pick. And the cycle continues. Uncomfortable emotions we want to avoid at all costs that we don't know what to do with. So we seek solace from ice cream, chocolate, and potato chips, or for others, these uncomfortable emotions may be comforted with alcohol or drugs. For me it was food. Always was.

After years and years of working with women, I have come to realize we're scared. We're scared to feel because once we do, we have no idea what is going to come up. And we are so scared of our own bodies that we don't listen. We don't trust it even when we do listen and notice. We don't love it for what it does for us. We have been taught just the opposite. We look at it, compare it, and contrast it to the latest photoshopped app, and we hate what we see. We feel aches, pains, bloating, fatigue—you name it, from our bodies, but ignore it. We just want to bury it all in the latest weight loss drug or treatment or surgery. Why are we so willing to cut, slash, and burn our bodies, yet so unwilling to pause, reflect, and listen to it; to ask it what message it is trying to send us?

So I've asked myself and wondered for other women: What exactly is going on physically, emotionally, and spiritually that we are so scared to look at? What are we so scared to feel? Are we so accustomed to not listening and not feeling because we may have to face something that is uncomfortable? Is there something we might have to change? The truth is, we are scared of our own bodies and how we feel because we've learned to suppress it all for so long and don't know what to do with its signals.

This realization that we're all suppressing so much and for so long was an epiphany for me because, in hindsight, I can see that I was no different. I was doing exactly that for years. I can look back now to a moment in my life where the anxiety I felt was debilitating and made me scared to leave my house. During this time, I was seeing my lifetime quota of doctors because no one knew how to help the dizziness, nausea, or fatigue that had over-taken my life one summer and kept me in my bed for months thereafter.

It was your typical hot August day in New York. I had gone for my usual run in the morning and distinctly told my husband when I came back, "I feel so frkn good!" Yet hours later my body literally collapsed and shut down. No warning. *Not really.* I had been suffering from severe bloating and thought nothing of it. On top of that, I had been stung by a bee in the beginning of the summer, and also thought nothing of that. And after that? Got into a little poison ivy playing ball with my kids. Again, thought nothing of any of it. But could they have been related? Could all of these situations that caused me to have inflammatory immune responses have been the tip of the iceberg for me? Was swimming in a local lake, and then showering in its waters, the driving force that finally put me over the edge— and into physical collapse— that summer morning? The truth is no one will ever know, yet in my heart of hearts, I do know there was a connection to it all. I didn't just collapse one day, without warning, without something causing it to happen.

I went from doctor to doctor. You name the specialist, I saw them. From vestibular therapists, neurologists, ENTs, endocrinologists, and general practitioners. Although all the practitioners were truly trying their best, in the short fifteen minutes they saw me, no one was closer to helping me. Bloodwork was drawn, and everything came up normal, except my thyroid. It was off, not crazy off to put me in bed for months, but off. So I went on the standard synthroid thyroid medication in hopes that would help.

It didn't.

And I knew no doctor would be able to help me. It wasn't their job. It was mine. But to appease my family, I continued to go from doctor to doctor. I think my family was more concerned about my state of health than I was then. You see, although I was very sick and felt terrible, I knew I would get better. There was never a doubt in my mind. I was not scared that I wouldn't get better, because I trusted I would. I just didn't know how, or when, but that I would get better was never a doubt in my mind. I had blind faith my body was doing what it needed to do. And it did. With a little help of course.

Every morning, after my husband went to work and my mother would get my children off to school, I would lay on the couch, in silence, meditating and envisioning my body healthy. I used essential oils. I took many supplements. I did breathwork. I reached out to work colleagues who were in the health field, and I put together my own plan of care—one that did not rely on medical intervention, but my own intervention. I had blind faith and leaned into the divine design of our beautiful bodies.

What brought me to this blind faith, to truly trust my body that it knew what it was doing, was not one particular moment, but the journey that began on the day I was called a blimp. My relationship with my body then was one of a nemesis. I would hate what I saw when I looked in the mirror. I would hate how I felt in my body. I would hate how it felt when people would look at me and I assumed they were thinking I was fat—a blimp. So I would stuff all those feelings down just to feel a sense of calm and control over my upset and hurt feelings. And my method of soothing myself, as mentioned, was food, which just perpetuated the cycle of self-loathing.

But then college came and my passion for nutrition and using food as medicine was lit. This fire inside me couldn't be put out. My body began to change. My mindset and my beliefs on how to achieve health, which was my personal priority, changed. It was innate—knowing that our bodies were brilliant. The icing on this realization of the wisdom of our body was the birth of my two daughters. With my first pregnancy I was so determined to have a natural childbirth, no epidural and no medical intervention. I was in labor for over 30 hours, pushed for five, and then when the doctors changed shifts, the new shift called for a Cesarean section. I was absolutely okay with that. I did my best to birth naturally, that just wasn't God's plan. My first daughter nursed like a champ right away. I was so proud. My second daughter was different. Once again I was determined to have a natural birth, but this time it was going against what was common for most. I was told to schedule a Cesarean section, but I said no. I had the desire and belief I could do it naturally. With the help and care of my midwife, this time I did. My daughter was born quickly and with a lot of blood loss from me. She was whisked away to the children's hospital and wasn't brought home for seven days. Yet I knew she would be fine. It was an uncanny knowing. It took over two weeks before she would nurse. Once again, I knew she would nurse and could nurse, I just needed to be patient and let what is a natural instinct in babies, and a natural process in my body, let it take its course. I did not give up. Needless to say, my second baby nursed for three years! Imagine if I had not learned and surrendered to the beautiful brilliance of our bodies? Learning to trust your body is a process we all can do. The birthing and nursing of my two daughters was the gift that cemented that deep trust in myself and my body.

That day in August when I collapsed? It wasn't about food then. It wasn't because I was stuffing my emotions down with food. But I also wasn't paying attention to my body just like I wasn't every time I over ate or ate when I wasn't actually hungry. I wasn't paying attention to the severe bloating. I wasn't actually listening to the signs and signals my body was giving me that summer and for many months before. So my body made me. In order to heal, I had to look at what was going on in my life that may have seemed overwhelming and where I wasn't digesting, or processing, my emotions so I could let them go.

I have come to realize that disease in the body is a physical manifestation of the mental and emotional ways that we are, either dealing or not dealing with, things in our life. It may start with stuffing our emotions down because we don't think we are meeting the external standards of beauty, as it did in my case. But if we don't stop this cycle of emotional suppression, we then eventually will see physical ailments. When we stuff our emotions down or judge our emotions, it keeps us from feeling, processing, and releasing them. Can we not look at our emotions as messengers without judgement—as a part of the beautiful way our body was designed to guide us?

We are humans with a wide range of emotions, but instead of feeling them, we have learned to shove them down or cut them off before they can release, and we spend years, or even decades, with them being trapped in our bodies. But these emotions are how our body communicates with us, so by suppressing our emotions we are suppressing the body's signs that we need to be listening to. When we don't, these long-suppressed emotions turn into physical ailments. For me, the result of suppressing so many emotions starting from the day I was called a blimp, resulted in my collapse that August morning followed by months of being unwell.

Instead of suppressing, ignoring, and possibly collapsing, let's meet our emotions with curiosity and reflection. What are the messages in them? Can we embrace them and not judge them and look to them as a gift for what they truly are? Can we welcome them and not resist them? Can we be present and feel, instead of running and cutting them out? Can we come from the ultimate place of unconditional love for ourselves, our bodies, and nurture and make our choices from that place instead? Can we learn to listen before the collapse?

And so my intention is to support and help women and our daughters release and let go of the things that we are carrying emotionally, mentally, and then ultimately, allow them to release physically, as well. We must listen to our body's nudges. We must trust that our body is the tuning fork and it will guide us like a true symphony.

The question then becomes: What if instead we saw our life perfect as-is, and loved ourselves, as-is, and had fun, as-is. And made all our decisions from a place of self love, not self loathing? What would our lives look like then?

So much of my life I waited to have fun—until I looked just right, had the perfect body, had enough money, had the perfect job. I kept putting off living my life fully until I had the perfect life and the perfect body. Guess what? "Perfect" never came.

I am grateful that I have learned to love and cherish my body as-is. Now. *Finally.* I don't want another daughter to lose the years I did, always wanting and waiting for the perfect day that everything perfectly falls into place and perfectly feels wonderful because that day will never come. I don't want another daughter to go their whole life searching on the outside for what is already given on the inside. I saw that with my own mom, always searching on the outside and never on inside, always stuffing the emotions and unease down. I saw it with the women at the gym, with my girlfriends, and the women in my extended family. And I saw it in myself. I never wanted to see it in my daughters.

I love days now.

I love how I look now. I love how I feel now. I go to the gym and I feel strength. I go not to change my body, although that is the effect. I go because I love my body. I have fun. It feels good to me. I get out of bed, and shuffle with early-morning achiness—sometimes it only takes a minute or two for the stiffness to go away. It's all good. I laugh to myself as I shuffle to the bathroom. I remember how my mom shuffled. My husband always said, "You're just like your mother." Thank God.

I only wish my mom could have seen the beautiful reflection of herself in the mirror. The one I saw as I watched her apply her makeup. I had the privilege of seeing her beauty inside and out.

I look in the mirror now and no longer want to hide. I love who I see in the mirror now more than ever. I no longer feel shame when I eat a brownie. I love putting makeup on. Because it's fun. And I like to wear no makeup too because I can. I see it all now. The crows feet around my eyes, the softness in my middle, the signs of aging on my skin. But gosh, I like who I see. Imagine if I felt this way twenty years ago?

I wish I had known then what I know now about emotions and my body. How to be okay with them and to listen, and then how to let them go in a way that serves your highest self. How to tap into the power of my heart. What a different place it is when you come from love of yourself and your body. But that was my lesson and now I am here to help others learn it too.

It is my greatest wish for all our daughters to know it's okay to feel all our emotions and then to process them and LET THEM GO. To know that suppressing our emotions may help us in the moment, but over time, the suppressing takes an emotional, mental, and physical toll on us.

Our health and happiness is an inside job. We have been led wrong. We have been led to look for outside sources and outside validation. But we have everything we need, if we just look within ourselves. Simply see the beauty in everything around us—in the sunset, in nature, in our children. All that beauty is reflected back to us, but it originates from within us.

How we love and see ourselves is how we will see the world, so the more beauty we can see within ourselves, the more beauty we'll see around us. Then we can start to see the beauty that is our bodies. We can see how much of a miracle the woman's body is to create life. What a wonder it is where we can start to notice how our legs can take us up mountains and how our arms can hold our loved ones. We can start to appreciate this body for the beauty that it allows us to experience in our world around us.

So it's time for us to come into a place where we no longer pinch our belly fat and say that we're too fat after just giving birth or we no longer judge one another for the shape or size of our bodies. The more beauty we see around us or within us is the more that can be reflected back to us.

Our highest potentials, our greatest gifts, can be realized when we begin to recognize our body's gentle guidance, to listen to our hearts and tap into its power, and let go of those feelings that no longer serve us. It is completely liberating. When we listen to our heart, we will never lose our way. When we listen to our heart, we go beyond the looking glass and love ourselves from the inside out.

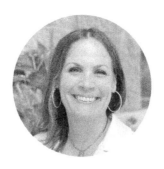

LAURA TOLOSI

Inspirational speaker, Integrative Nutritionist and No-Diet Weight Loss Coach for women with 30+ years experience. Specializing in physical and emotional metabolism, Laura Tolosi, known as The Diet Ditcher, is on a quest to help women of all ages fall in love with their bodies from a place of self love and self worth.

Laura's passion is for all women to be confident in their bodies while enjoying food that nourishes and tastes good without feeling guilt or shame. Her signature Emotional Metabolism Method helps women tap into the power of their heart and the innate wisdom of their body.

Her ultimate mission is for women to go beyond the looking glass and love themselves from the inside out. You can reach Laura via email at: Laura@lauratolosinutrition.com.

Within the moment where it feels as if our life trajectory has changed forever, we can pause and come into a place of acceptance for what is so that we can truly move forward with beauty and grace.

CHAPTER NINE

Beautiful Chaos

Written by Miranda Pellett

When I look over my life up until this moment in time, there are two words that I feel perfectly describe my experience: *Beautiful Chaos*. As I sit to write this chapter, which really is a journey into my oldest daughter's diagnosis and all that came with it, I'm realizing that even though you may not have this exact storyline playing out in your life, I am sure at one point or another, each of us have experienced traumas, losses, hardships, or challenges that have made us realize that our life—the life that we planned for, dreamt of, that we thought was going to be our future, how it was inevitably going to play out, is not in fact, what we have experienced. But there is an opportunity here; an opportunity that within that moment where it feels as if our life trajectory has changed forever, that we can pause and we can find that as we grieve the future that we thought was ours, we can come into a place of acceptance for what is and forgetting what was, so that we can truly move forward with beauty and grace.

As a young girl, really my whole life, I have suffered with social anxiety, though when I was younger, "anxiety" in children was never really talked about—definitely not as much as it is today. Back when I was young it was simply labeled as being shy, or antisocial, but it would manifest in ways where I couldn't cross the street if someone was walking on the other side. I couldn't go to the park unless I had my younger sister with me giving me a sense of comfort, safety, and security. Even as a teenager, I couldn't call and order a pizza; I would freeze and hang up as soon as the person answered.

After years of infertility, I finally became a mom for the first time, and my anxiety ramped up even further. I remember holding my daughter, Ameliya, in my arms at our home in the birthing tub and though there was this feeling of immense love and gratitude, with it came this deep sense of fear and soon after, a debilitating sense of anxiety. When I knew someone was coming over to visit and meet our daughter, I would sit and sob at the mere thought of someone else holding her. I would stay in the nursery, rocking in the chair, and crying until my husband brought Ameliya back into my arms. There was always this deep sense of dread and fear that something bad was going to happen to my daughter. They called it postpartum anxiety and labeled it as something irrational telling me nothing was going to happen. And yet it was as if I was just fearing an experience happening before it did; a premonition of Ameliya's life and what was to come.

I remember Ameliya being eighteen months old, and it being the first time that I had allowed my husband to take her in a vehicle without me. As I watched them drive away, tears started to flow and they didn't stop until the car pulled back in the driveway three hours later, with Ameliya safe and sound. I had been overcome by intrusive thoughts that something bad was going to happen to Ameliya when she was out of my care. I could never shake the thoughts and feelings, no matter how hard I tried. What's interesting about this situation is that when Ameliya was twenty-two months old, we welcomed our second daughter, Clara, into the world and our family, and everything with her was completely different. Within a couple weeks of Clara being born I was able to leave her with my sister while Ameliya and I went grocery shopping, and I was able to do that with no fear or anxiety. It wasn't that I loved Clara any less than Ameliya, I just never had any hesitation about her safety. There was a sense of calm and peace knowing she would be fine. It's interesting looking back at the difference between the two girls and how I handled them as newborns and knowing that my anxiety was helping to keep me alert and aware as I was sensing something intuitively.

When Ameliya was two and a half years old, she was a happy and healthy toddler, running around, dancing everywhere she went, playing soccer and gymnastics, and loving on her baby sister. It was September 2016 and Ameliya had developed a respiratory virus, just a simple cold that had been going through our extended family. The cold only lasted a few days and soon enough she was back to her energetic self and attending her gymnastics class on Saturday, as per usual that fall. However, a few hours after this particular gymnastics class I noticed Ameliya starting to limp around the house. I asked my husband if something happened at gymnastics and he said no, not that he had seen. I thought that perhaps she had stepped on one of the many toys scattered around the house and she would be fine. The next day I noticed that this limp had gotten a bit worse in that she would fall after taking a couple steps. She would get back up, take a few more steps and fall. I feared she had done something at gymnastics that needed to be looked at more closely and said I would take her to our chiropractor the next day. By the next morning, she was no longer able to take steps without holding onto something, so I immediately made the appointment with our chiropractor and he got us in right away that Monday morning. After looking her leg over he didn't sense anything was severely wrong and suggested she rest, alternate ice and heat, and that if it got worse, to take her to the hospital. By the time my husband got home from work that evening Ameliya was only able to crawl, with her right leg dragging behind her. I knew something was severely wrong, so we called our pediatrician and had her meet us at our local emergency room. She ran blood work and X-rays on Ameliya and after seven hours overnight in the hospital, along with Clara who was seven months old at the time, they had no answers for us. Both the on-call doctor and our pediatrician figured she must have suffered from a toddler fracture that wasn't showing on the X-rays. They sent us home saying to continue giving her pain medication and lots of rest. In my gut I knew something wasn't right, but who was I to argue with professional medical advice? *I'm just a mom.*

That next day (Tuesday), my mom had taken the day off to help me with the kids as we had been in the hospital all night and were exhausted. I vividly remember sitting at my computer in the kitchen and looking up Ameliya's symptoms online; *I would highly suggest not doing this—nothing good ever comes from "Dr. Google."* The first diagnosis to pop up was leukemia. *I lost it.* I called my husband at work and told him to meet us at CHEO (Children's Hospital of Eastern Ontario) in Ottawa, a large children's hospital an hour from where we lived. Upon arrival I didn't know what to expect; but I certainly didn't expect to be sent home a few hours later. In fact, I was relieved! Transient synovitis is what the emergency on-call doctors had diagnosed Ameliya with—a common hip irritant in children that typically follows an ailment or virus. It all made sense—she would be back to her happy and energetic, fully mobile self within the week. *Or so we thought.*

Sitting around and waiting for your two-year-old toddler to start walking on their own again is excruciating. Every night I would go to bed and pray that by the next morning I would be awoken by Ameliya running into my bedroom and jumping on the bed like she had done every morning prior to her illness. Wednesday would come and go, and all Ameliya did was sleep. We had a follow-up appointment with her pediatrician that day who also agreed with CHEO's diagnosis of transient synovitis. Thursday came and went and there was no forward progression. I remember sitting on the floor playing with both girls and Ameliya had fallen asleep while playing, except she didn't fall asleep lying backwards, she fell asleep lying on her side across my leg. I remember thinking her positioning was strange; I even have a picture I took of this very moment that I've looked back on numerous times since.

Friday, October 6, 2016, was the day that I decided to step up and advocate for my daughter on a whole other level. It was also the day that our entire lives, and that of our future lives, were completely flipped upside down. Trying to give Ameliya breakfast that morning, she could no longer hold her spoon to feed herself yogurt. I knew right away that this had now gone above the hip. *Her diagnosis was wrong.* Once again, I called my mom and my husband and told them to meet us at CHEO. We were going back, and I wasn't going to leave that hospital until someone could tell me what was wrong with my daughter. Upon getting the two girls in their car seats it was the first time that Ameliya had really indicated any pain the entire week. She couldn't sit in her car seat without screaming in pain. I contemplated calling an ambulance; I just needed to get my daughter to the hospital. I ended up switching her car seat from rear-facing to forward-facing, and putting the movie Tangled (Rapunzel) on the van's DVD entertainment system. It was enough to get her calmed down and distracted so that I could drive to Ottawa. I distinctly remember the look on my husband's face when he looked back to Ameliya and saw that her head was now lying on her shoulder. She no longer had the ability or strength to hold her head up. We looked at each other with fear in our eyes, but no words. Neither of us wanted to say anything; *we were both fearing the worst.*

Thankfully this trip to the emergency department at CHEO saw us with a neurologist as the on-call doctor. He ran a few quick tests with Ameliya there on the bed, looked at me and said, "You need to make arrangements with your husband and younger daughter, because Ameliya isn't going to be leaving this hospital anytime soon." *My heart sank.* It was confirmation that something was seriously wrong. We were quickly admitted into the hospital and as it was nearly two in the morning, my husband

and Clara were given a room across the road at the Rotel; a small motel typically used by families who have children at CHEO. I was exclusively breastfeeding Clara at the time and so not only was my oldest daughter going through an emergency health situation, but this was also now the first night I was spending away from our baby. The hospital continued running tests on Ameliya throughout the night, including X-rays, CT scan, and an MRI with contrast. Nothing was coming up positive for any type of diagnosis. During those tests, I had many doctors coming to speak with me, trying to go back through Ameliya's history and what had happened the week(s) prior to her sudden illness. A student doctor came at one point and explained to me that it's like the medical TV show, House, where they have a big whiteboard with possible diagnoses on it and as each one gets ruled out, they cross it out and try the next one. So many doctors in such a short amount of time. I even still feel anger when I remember a conversation with one of the first neurologists I spoke to that Friday night. I had gone through everything that had happened that week, all her symptoms and she said to me, "So this started last Saturday and you're just now bringing her in?" *I saw red.* We had been to multiple hospitals, that one included, seen and talked to many doctors who had run numerous tests, and Ameliya was continuously misdiagnosed, making us feel like Ameliya's condition wasn't serious. In fact, one doctor suggested Ameliya was faking her symptoms to gain the attention of her parents. I wasn't being heard, no one was listening to me. Everything felt like it was being swept under the rug and not being given the attention it deserved. But this was my child, and I was done with not being heard. That night we were finally heard. With it being Thanksgiving weekend, I was told that many doctors were off and that the tests needing to be done may have to wait until after the long weekend. Absolutely not! My daughter's life was on the line; I didn't care who they needed to call to run the final test, but they needed to get there, and it needed to be done now. By breakfast that next morning, Ameliya was being taken down for a lumbar puncture (spinal tap), and that's where they found the elevated protein levels in the spinal fluid, giving her a diagnosis of Guillain-Barre Syndrome (GBS). *We finally had an answer.*

Guillain-Barre Syndrome (Ghee-yan Bah-ray) is a rare autoimmune disease defined by the rapid onset of numbness, weakness, and often paralysis of the legs, arms, breathing muscles, and face. It's an inflammatory disorder of the peripheral nerves outside the brain and spinal cord. The cause of GBS is unknown but it is said that a majority of cases occur shortly after a microbial infection (viral or bacterial), some as simple and common as the flu or food poisoning. GBS causes damage to the myelin sheath (nerve covering), leading to numbness and weakness typically starting in the toes and ascending upwards. There is no cure for GBS; however, most patients are given IVIG (Intravenous Immune Globulins) in high doses or plasma exchange (a blood "cleansing") to shorten the course of the acute phase. This phase can vary in length from a few days to months. The majority of patients will be admitted to the Intensive Care Unit for their breathing to be monitored as GBS can cause paralysis to reach the lungs and diaphragm, forcing the patient to be put on a ventilator to breathe.

GBS is rare, 2 in 100,000 people, but even more rare in children of Ameliya's age. It was never even close to being on the radar when doctors were looking at her in the week prior and therefore led to multiple misdiagnoses. We would spend twenty days in the hospital; her dad and I switching off in the evenings so that I could spend the night with Clara across the road at Ronald McDonald House. During that time Ameliya would go through many tests to determine how much damage was done to her body and what the prognosis might be. GBS survivors can typically regain the majority of their mobility and strength back within one year; however, the results of nerve conduction studies done on Ameliya would diagnose her further with the GBS variant AMAN (acute motor axonal neuropathy). Not only was the myelin sheath around the peripheral nerves damaged but so were the axons themselves. We soon learned that this would result in permanent nerve damage in both of Ameliya's legs.

My little girl, who I envisioned going to dance classes, playing soccer, and participating in swimming lessons... There was an overwhelming sense of grief when we got the prognosis. Grieving this future that I thought would be hers; feeling as if she wouldn't be able to have the whole life experience like I had hoped for her, like we hope as mothers for our children. And so, there was this piece of me that could go down this negative spiral of what I could have done differently to prevent this horrible situation, but I know that is a spiral we don't want to get sucked into. What's done is done; the path that we walked is walked. No matter what situation you find yourself in or are trying to navigate, we must come to full acceptance of what is now in this present moment.

As I look back at this experience and I see Ameliya now at ten years old, she is walking with a mobility walker and braces on her legs, but she's also dancing, playing soccer, and swimming—it just looks a little different. I believe that there are so many lessons that Ameliya and my own experience can teach us all. We need to trust our intuition above all else, above any "degreed" person, or anyone with any number of professional letters behind their name. We need to understand that our intuition can guide us to the truth. We need to listen, and we need to stop putting our power and our life in other's hands. We need to have the courage to advocate for ourselves and for those who are not able to advocate for themselves. We need to stop taking no for an answer when we know that we need a yes, in whatever circumstance or situation. We need to have the courage to speak up, demand better, and continue to question everything. We need to also understand and realize that the trajectory of our life can completely change in a single moment.

I never could have imagined that right now I would be sitting here writing this chapter at thirty-eight years old, a recently separated and now single mom with four young children, ages ten, eight, five, and three, and doing it on my own. And yet through it all, it has made me stronger. Life events like this show us who we are and what we're made of.

As I look at Ameliya, I see the strength she has, the ability for her to be different, and to learn to own who she is. For her to say, I'm going to dance anyway and then do it; the resilience that this experience is teaching her and for all future experiences yet to come in her life. There's no other way she could have received that level of strength and resilience. Though life can hand us things that change the course of our life forever, we can also find the glimmer of hope within it; the gift, and the lesson in it all. Ultimately, what I believe is the greatest gift that this has taught us all is how to live in the beautiful chaos. Life is not perfect. We can't control everything. There are going to be moments of trauma and change and loss and hardship because that's life. We don't always get to decide or choose when those challenges happen; it comes as a shock, it comes out of nowhere, a complete blind side. Yet often we have been preparing for these big moments in life, we just maybe didn't fully understand or see the bigger picture. And when those moments come, yes, they feel devastating, but we must walk the path of anger and grief, and ultimately, acceptance and peace, knowing that we did all we could with the best that we had, and knowing and trusting that we can move forward no matter what and that we will be stronger for it. We need to come to terms with the idea that life is really a series of chaotic moments, but there is always beauty to be found in them, if only we are open and willing to see it.

Accept what is, let go of what was, and have faith in what will be.
– Sonia Ricotti

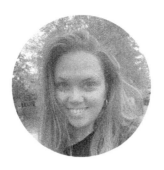

MIRANDA PELLETT

Miranda Pellett is a devoted solo mom to four young children living in a small town in Eastern Ontario, Canada. Her strong passion for Christmas, baking, walking along the St. Lawrence River, and reading are just a few things that she loves to fill her time with outside of her busy mom schedule. After her daughter Ameliya's life altering diagnosis in 2016, advocacy for accessibility also joined that list. Miranda volunteers as a patient communication liaison for the GBS/CIDP Foundation of Canada where she communicates with other families and helps to support young children after diagnosis. Miranda, along with her daughter Ameliya, won the 2023 Walter Keast Award for all of their work with the foundation raising money to support critical care programs and increasing GBS awareness. In 2023 Miranda spoke at the International GBS-CIDP Symposium in Washington, DC of her journey with Ameliya's diagnosis. She looks forward to continuing to raise awareness through speaking engagements in the future and is also looking forward to expanding her chapter and writing a full-length book on her daughter's journey to walk again. You can connect with Miranda through Instagram @mama24miracles or email mpellett@gbscidp.ca.

I'm still her.

CHAPTER TEN

Go Back to the Beginning

Written by Paula Campbell

Throughout my life, I have always gone back to the beginning. In the most challenging of times, I go back to my childhood. When we were young, we were innocent and imaginative. We didn't care about what others thought. There weren't any obstacles in our way. We only saw adventure! We had no worries because that wasn't our job. Our job was to be a kid.

Who would have thought that our younger self could teach us so much as we got older? We see where all the quirky traits came from. We see where the daydreaming started. And as we grow, we see where those very dreams became broken and where we kept getting the same lessons over and over again, until finally—hopefully, we learned them. We learn that our biggest wake up calls come from our experiences and the opportunity for growth lies in our reactions and our actions.

As a child, I started out carefree and creative. I could keep myself entertained for hours. I loved being outside as a kid. One of my favorite things to do was to play "make believe." I was so fascinated by the movie, *Wizard of Oz*. I would dress up and pretend I was Dorothy and take my dog in the field behind our house and go on an adventure. My friend down the street would meet me and play the Scarecrow. There was an old barn in the field and we pretended it was the house that fell on the witch. We had it all figured out. I could escape any part of the real world by living in this make-believe one for a few hours. I loved the idea of this girl finding her way on her own, yet meeting different strangers along the way. She was scared and wanted to find her way back and thought she needed to see the wizard to get her home, but really she had the answers within her the whole time.

I was so intrigued by this story and saw it as a grand adventure. There are so many hidden messages in that movie. Going back to that memory reminds me of my younger self, the carefree, imaginative girl that created an adventure in her backyard. The girl who could feel insecure at times but used her sense of humor to get her through the most uncertain times.

Years later when I became a teenager, there were parts of me that wanted to go back to the days in elementary school where everything was simple, but high school is a little tougher. It's not a gradual process between the two, you go from one place to a completely different one and it happens quickly. We aren't allowed to be the same. We aren't kids anymore. It's like your childhood is in fast-forward mode and now you have to face this new experience all the while remembering who you once were. You start to meet new friends but try to keep the old ones from your childhood for just a little bit longer, all the while curious about new experiences. It's easy to lose yourself in those years as insecurities take hold.

High school requires optimism, yet a need to be guarded and cautious. Friendships and interactions can be natural or complicated. My teen years were tricky at times. I got caught up in the social part of being a teenager and stopped trying in my classes. I didn't really know what I was good at or what I enjoyed anymore because I started to lose myself. I found it hard to concentrate in school because of other things that were going on and I started to fall behind. I can look back now and see I was growing up and it's a process that's not always easy. My experiences led to some mistakes but those mistakes led to wake-up calls. Once I reached my twenties and got through more hard times, I looked back at my teen years and thought those years of my life didn't matter anymore, it wasn't really me; it was just a time in my life when I was struggling to figure things out. I wasn't focused on what was important at that time because, like Dorothy, I didn't know how to get there on my own. I felt misunderstood and needed guidance. Looking back now as an adult, I wish I had someone to help me through that time. That's probably why I'm so drawn to helping others now. I've always been an empathetic person, so perhaps I needed to go through darker times in order to truly help people now.

After high school, I kept bouncing ideas around about what I wanted to do with my life. I had several jobs and worked full time but I wanted more for myself. I would go to night school and take classes that I needed for potential university programs, but I wouldn't follow through. I continued to sabotage myself by procrastinating. I felt eager and ready to tap into my interests, yet I wouldn't stick with it. I kept allowing other things to get in the way of my dreams. I yearned to do something I was good at and I wanted to make a difference in whatever career I had. But I just kept getting in my own way.

I would have become a nutritionist or had a job in social work or broadcasting if I followed through with any of it. It's interesting how much you change as you get older but how you stay true to certain interests. I've been into fitness and nutrition since I was eighteen and I'm still intrigued by it now. Throughout my life, I have regretted not pursuing my interests and I'd be lying if I said it didn't torment me for years. But by the time I thought I knew what I wanted to do, there were different plans for me.

When I was eighteen, I lost both my grandfathers. Not long after I lost my first Grandpa in March, I developed an allergic reaction that would become a battle for years to come, but later that year, at 19 I entered into a relationship that was quite difficult. When everyone my age was going out and having fun, I was in a supportive role to someone who was struggling with addiction. I went to meetings to support this person, but the stronger I tried to be, the more fragile I became. I started to lose myself more by the day. This experience made it hard for me to trust people, which was a struggle after I eventually moved on. I had become codependent, wanting to be supportive but I lost myself in the process. I felt myself slipping away from who I wanted to be, so far away from the little girl who so confidently found adventures. Shortly after this person sought treatment, I was in my first month at a new job at a beer and wine store. During one of my shifts I was robbed at knifepoint. This was one of the most terrifying experiences I'd had in my life. I remember the way he made small talk with me before he came to the counter and told me to give him the money. That's when I saw the knife, as he raised it up towards me. The counter was waist height, so there wasn't much space in between us. I remember feeling like I couldn't breathe. The room was blurry and his eyes were dark. I was having a panic attack. He took what money I had and told me to sit on the floor and count back from one hundred. It is in these moments you ask yourself if this is really happening? *How did I end up here?* Anxiety filled my body.

As I faced the wall, sitting cross legged on the floor, I stopped counting when I felt he had left and I called 911. I don't remember what I said. I proceeded to lock myself in the bathroom, where I stared at my ghostly face in the mirror. It was an out of body experience. I didn't feel connected to myself at all. I was looking at myself having this experience but I had no control over my mind and body. I saw my reflection in the mirror and didn't recognize who was looking back at me.

After giving my statement to the police, I drove home, where I still lived with my parents and casually told my dad what happened. I was grateful that he was the only one home because his reaction was caring but calm, therefore I had no one feeding my anxiety. I went back to work the next day because I knew if I didn't, it would haunt me. I had to jump back in or I would become numb by this situation. By going back to work the next day, it made me put one foot in front of the other. *Keep going, you are okay.*

When I had to pick the robber out of a photo lineup, I had the exact same feeling in my stomach that I had that day. His photo stuck out to me because his face became blurry and his eyes became dark, my body was numb. I knew it was him. I had to attend court and I was put on the stand. Everyone knew I was a victim in this but the perpetrator's lawyer treated me like I was the criminal. I guess that's his job to protect his client, but I was an innocent twenty-two year old that just suffered something traumatic. I felt alone, yet I was told by another lawyer I should feel privileged to experience a courtroom. "What a jerk," I thought.

After I testified in court, I did what most young people do, I tried to move on and forget about it. At least I thought I moved on until I would find myself numb at times by the slightest trigger that reminded me of that day. I would spend the next several years experiencing numbing anxiety and panic attacks but it took me years to figure out why it was happening. I was suffering from PTSD. I would hide it but inside I was a mess.

When we experience something traumatic we push it out of our mind and try to forget, but the body remembers. The body reminds you, there are still some things you need to heal from. I eventually left that job to find one that was less triggering for me.

By now my allergic reactions that started when I was eighteen had become a real nuisance in my life. I would miss weeks of work because my face would be swollen. My body would be covered in a rash and no one could help me. I was given the same excuses from doctors. It's an allergic reaction, it will pass. "You'll grow out of it!" It didn't make any sense, because I didn't have reactions like this before, so why now? It had to be more than a skin reaction. I started to believe our emotions create havoc in our bodies and there were years of emotions trying to surface and those emotions were coming out through my skin. Doctors gave me steroid creams and allergy shots, Prednisone, and so on. I can't count how many times I drove to the emergency department to get an allergy shot in hopes it would take away the swelling. I became depressed. Doctors couldn't figure it out, so I decided to see what I could find out on my own. I became interested in nutrition and cleanses and even took Reiki classes. I was determined to figure out why this was happening.

The healing world, at this time, was filled with people far older than me. I would go to people's houses and learn Reiki in a room full of strangers. We would learn from a Reiki master by practicing on anyone that would volunteer. It was a calm atmosphere, filled with like-minded people who believed in the power of healing.

I tried meditation in hopes it would help me to stop overthinking. I would go to different places where they held meditation sessions and found myself lying on the floor amongst strangers trying to find a peaceful place in my mind. Quieting my thoughts was always hard for me. I was always worrying and always thinking, I couldn't shut my mind off. I lived in "what if" mode and it was exhausting, and the insomnia I suffered for so long hadn't helped. I often wondered if I was experiencing anxiety from not sleeping or if I was not sleeping because of the anxiety. The older me looks back and thinks anxiety was a reaction to the worried thoughts and the worries led to not sleeping and round and round it went, one causing the other and the other becoming worse. We need calm and we need sleep for survival—I had neither. I wasted years researching insomnia when I really should have been focusing on things that helped me feel calm. I really should have followed my instincts instead of doing things I didn't want to do. I was restless because I wasn't living a life authentic to who I wanted to be.

I continued to have skin reactions that were quite debilitating. I would wake up with a swollen face and swollen joints. My eyes were often swollen shut. There was a stressful point in my life where I developed psoriasis on my scalp but thankfully it went away after that particular part of my life passed. Our skin is our biggest organ and mine was definitely trying to tell me something. I didn't know what I was waking up to each day and it was a sign I couldn't ignore. I had to find out why. Why was my body overreacting to everything in sight? I remember meeting Rosa Gee at Health Harmony Healing Centre. Rosa specialized in acupuncture, colonic treatment and Chinese medicine. She was so kind to me and made me feel so hopeful. She would speak of cleansing the body of toxins but also cleansing the body of old emotions.

I would go to see Rosa weekly for several years. People like Rosa were mentors to me on my healing journey. She educated me on healing my body from toxins—physically and mentally.

I started to see a naturopath who I still see today. I have been his patient for thirty years and I have to say I consider him a long time friend. I get so much from these appointments, even now. He is a wiseman and a healer to many. He helped me by looking at how to get my body balanced. My allergic reaction was not something I was going to grow out of; something was off and I had to fix it. I started drinking green drinks every morning, eating clean, taking probiotics, and reading any self-help book I could.

I found books by Lousie Hay and started to see the power of thought which has become quite well known today. Positive thinking is all over social media and the Internet now, yet Louise Hay is really the one who started affirmations. She was fifty years old when she made a pamphlet called, "Heal Your Body", that was later enlarged and extended into her first book, *You Can Heal Your Life.* This was the first book I read by Louise Hay. She was 58 years old when she published it. *You Can Heal Your Life* was about the power of our thoughts and how we have the power to change our circumstances by starting with how we think. She connected thoughts to the disease and affirmations to the healing. This book was the starting point to learning the concept of "you become what you think."

We attract our circumstances without even knowing it. We can change the way we think at any given time, so why do we choose self-defeating thoughts instead of encouraging ones?

I became so hopeful by reading books and seeing natural healers. I found a natural doctor, Dr. Cline, who not only identified the problem, he helped me get my body balanced. I was a business teller at the bank and his wife would bring in the deposits. One day she noticed I had been away for a while and asked where I had been. I told her about my allergic reactions and she said her husband was having a seminar on allergies and recommended I come. I went to the seminar and finally got the answers I was looking for. Allergies are an imbalance in your immune system, so I needed to figure where the imbalance was. Dr. Cline said everything starts in the gut, so we started there with probiotics and acidophilus, along with other vitamins and then changed my diet.

Dr. Cline was the turning point for me. If I hadn't started to see Dr

Cline or my naturopath, I would have continued seeing traditional doctors and gotten nowhere. I am unsure if I ever would have gotten any answers or seen any real results, never mind actually healed. I had been prescribed Prednisone for several years and took all kinds of prescriptions and anti-histamines, which are hard on your body over time. Not only was I not healing, my body was being battered with these medicines.

While I was taking control of my health, the allergic reactions would lessen but when they did arise I changed *my* reaction to them. Instead of panicking and feeling hopeless, I'd start to tell myself it would be okay and reverse the worried thoughts. I found the skin reactions weren't as bad or wouldn't last as long when I changed my reaction. I continued to eat healthy and take my vitamins. I continued to read self-help books and books on health. I went to yoga and hiked on weekends. I found that working out was the best medicine for my mind and it helped to quiet my thoughts and I slept better. I can honestly say that exercise changed me. When I run, I only think of positive things. When I'm walking on trails, I only think of creative ideas and I find the answers to what I am looking for. When I move my body and honor myself by taking the time to show up, I become stronger and wiser each time. Exercise is medicine. I crave it, I love it, and I am so grateful for it!

I spent a few years on my own, working and sticking to exercise and healthy eating. I educated myself by reading books on mind and body con-nection and living a pretty healthy lifestyle.

Life got more comfortable because I got more comfortable with myself. Whenever the anxiety rolled in, I had the tools to push it back out. I was in between where I wanted to be and where I was still figuring things out, but I wasn't completely lost anymore. I was starting to get my old self back. The little girl who loved adventure and the little girl who wanted to find something exciting came back to me again, so I would get off work and head to the trails knowing it always felt like an adventure.

Friendships faded and new ones came along. It was a time of change but always felt like everything was meant to be. Friendships were the one thing that came and went with a sense of ease. I had the right friends in my life when I needed them. It's interesting how you meet the right people at the right times. When I met someone who struggled with addiction, I met several co-workers who were recovering. I got their perspective and then I was able to support other people down the road because of my experience.

A few years later, I met my husband and life started happening fast. He saw life in fast forward which was a tad startling but also good for my procrastinating mind. For the first time in a long time, I felt cared for and admired. We became inseparable and life started moving quickly. Sure, he had a dog that I was allergic to and the dog was a maniac, but we got through it. We got engaged after a year. We married after two years and had our first son two years after getting married. My husband really wanted to start his own logging company, so we took the leap. We had our son in June and started a company the following March.

A year and a half later we had our second son. My husband never stopped planning the next move. We had two young boys and were trying to build a company and decided it was a good time to build a house. It was chaotic and stressful at times but life moves fast, so we had to make some big decisions. Neither one of us knew anything about running a business, but we learned along the way. We continued to grow the company, while raising our two sons and I don't regret a moment of it. It was a grind but I believed in my husband's big ideas and it turns out he knew what he was doing because it's twenty years later and the company is still running.

Our two boys are grown now. Raising my kids gave me back my childhood over and over again. I got to witness their innocence, curiosity, and creative young minds grow. I experienced laughter and saw imagination at its best. I had the best company with every story book we read and had the pleasure of watching them play sports and meet amazing new friends in the process. I got to enjoy watching them be themselves wholeheartedly, without a care in the world.

All those years in my twenties, thirties, and forties when I felt unworthy by not having my own career, only to look back now and see I had the best job in the world. There is nothing better than being a mother. Over the years I've learned that once you experience the beautiful things in life, you realize the hard times were only ever there to make you stronger. Life can be hard, yes, but once the tough times pass, we all walk away differently. There's always something greater ahead, we just don't see it until we get there.

But, it all works out eventually, doesn't it? All the times I felt lost and helpless and all the times I couldn't find my voice and didn't feel good enough and felt I was going nowhere. I see now that, somehow, it just works out. Everything works out eventually. Through it all I've learned to be true to myself and to stay in today. It took me years but I've finally let go of all those worried thoughts and the anxiety and insomnia it brought me. I healed myself when I stopped living in the "what if" mindset and partnered with healing modalities and practitioners that helped me most. The regrets and dwelling on the past were getting me nowhere. I needed everything I experienced so that I could get to the place where I have my beautiful life.

I have learned throughout my life that I am a strong person. If I have moments of weakness or feel anxious, I know what to do now. I know who I am and I remember that creative, imaginative little girl I once was. The girl who got lost on an adventure and found her way back home. I'm still her.

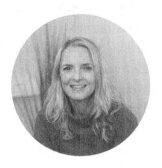

PAULA CAMPBELL

Paula Campbell lives on Vancouver Island. She finds motivation from being with like-minded positive people who share the same interests, whether that be at work or in life. Paula's love for people is what brought her to writing in this series. She loves stories and learning about other people's adventures. Her dream is to become a writer and seek out new possibilities because it's never too late for a new adventure. You can connect with Paula through email at p-campbell@shaw.ca.

I thought I would be broken forever; but luckily that was not true.

Sensitivity Advisory: This chapter references personal experiences of death of a spouse.

CHAPTER ELEVEN

Life After A Death

Written by Elaine De Rooy

It was just after midnight when the telephone rang. At first I thought it was in my dream but it didn't stop. I finally realized it was the phone beside the bed. I was disoriented at first. I had only fallen asleep a few hours ago and I was in a strange place—a hotel room in Vancouver booked just that afternoon. I groggily answered the phone and immediately wished I never had to hear what was said to me. My husband was dead. In a heartbeat, I was no longer a wife; I was a widow.

I was only sixteen years old when I met my husband for the first time. My best friend at the time was dating his roommate. I tagged along one time to their apartment. He was there getting ready for work. He was working the afternoon shift at the local paper mill, as a paper maker. I can't say it was love at first sight, but I do remember moments of that visit, which I used to use as a reason why I kept my eye on him after that encounter. He was eating Kraft Dinner out of a pot, with ketchup no less! Believing myself to be not that good of a cook at the time, I thought to myself: here is a man that isn't a picky eater, he might make a good man to tolerate my less-than-stellar cooking.

He was dating someone else at the time, so my story is that I bided my time. The truth was, I was young and inexperienced with men and dating. He went through two girlfriends before I had a shot at the title. I even told the story jokingly about having one of them deported back to Finland in order to clear the field for myself. The fact is that she was here with her family, and left and went back home with them, but I liked to tell two versions of the story. The funny one followed by the true one, on how my husband and I got together.

We met again, when his roommate started dating my older sister.

Yes we lived in a small town, where there were only so many eligible men around. At that time, he was unattached. At first he was reluctant to date me, because of the roommate connection. I must have won him over with my charm and intellect, since back then, I didn't consider myself to be much of a "looker." Our first date didn't go well, it involved the police pulling us over, poor recordkeeping at the police station, and my parents coming to our rescue. But as luck would have it, he was resilient, I was understanding, and we were married five years later.

At first, we had decided not to have children. Then my sister sent me all these craft Christmas ornaments. I used to do them on my lunch break at work. I called them my four hundred dollar ornaments since I worked in an accounting office and that was my charge-out rate for the number of hours I spent on each one. When I had finished the last one, I looked at my end result, and came to the realization that all my hard work was for nothing if I didn't have anyone to pass them onto. I managed to convince my husband to have children, on the explicit agreement that we have two, and not just one. I don't know why he wanted two, but I am glad he did. My two boys, or should I say men, have given me more pleasure over the years than the eighteen months of combined discomfort and pain they caused me in bringing them into the world.

We were a pretty typical family trying to juggle work, family, and personal time. My two boys were into the usual boy things—soccer, scouts, cadets. We went on family vacations to Mexico almost every year. My youngest was a pool water baby, and the oldest loved to ocean body surf.

Then in one instant all our lives were shattered and thrown aside. My husband, their father, had a sudden cardiac arrest while working out at a local gym. That fact that he was in a gym and not where we planned he be saved his life, for the moment.

He was supposed to be bike riding with our sons that evening, but instead decided to go workout to relieve some pent up stress from a busy day. During his workout, he decided to stop to rehydrate at the water fountain. That was the moment that his body lost control, and his heart started to beat too fast. He collapsed, and was kept alive by CPR performed by other gym members. The ambulance arrived and had to perform several shocks to bring his heart back into a somewhat regular rhythm. He was rushed to our local hospital.

I vividly remember being mad at him that evening for changing the family plan since I had to take the kids biking instead of him. To this day I distinctly remember hearing his ambulance while we were biking without realizing at the time that he was in it.

As my children and I were approaching our house after our bike ride, we saw an unfamiliar van parked in the driveway with the motor running, and no one inside. I was immediately on high alert, since we had been burglarized not that long ago. I told the kids to stay in the front yard, and I planned on confronting the individual, with my maternal instincts in full gear. When I realized who was at my house, I was confused at first. It was the owner of the local gym. She told me what happened. I really don't remember the details of what I did next. What I do remember was calling my parents to come take care of my boys, and then driving to the hospital.

At some point I called my younger sister, a registered nurse, to come to the hospital to be with me. She was there for most of the discussions regarding my husband's condition. I remember being totally overwhelmed by the whole experience, and grateful to have her there to explain what the doctor's were saying—in layman's terms. He was kept in hospital for quite some time and was subjected to many tests to determine his diagnosis. In the end, they could not determine a cause, just the result, problems with his heart.

After a heart angiogram, he was told that there was nothing wrong with his "pipes," but there was a problem with his "electrical." His upper heart, that was supposed to control his rhythm, was weakened, and that left the lower part of his heart, to figure out the pacing—and it wasn't doing a very good job at that. The answer was a pacemaker/defibrillator unit, which was implanted near his heart under his skin. This unit created some interesting issues in his life. It could go off at any moment if it detected an irregular heartbeat and it was made of metal, so proved challenging when we went on a vacation that involved traveling by air through airport security.

When he was still in hospital, I had an internal conflict between wanting to be with my children through all this and wanting to be by his side—to be his voice, since he had no memory of what happened to him. To this day, I wish I could somehow have been in both places at once since I know my kids were traumatized as much as I was by all the uncertainty surrounding his health.

He recovered slowly from the cardiac arrest, and things seemed to return to a somewhat normal routine. But that was not to last. He started experiencing decline in his health a few years later. Luckily we'd had a chance to go on a few vacations together as a family, and just the two of us, before his health really deteriorated.

His health decline looked like steps. It would drop, then level out, then drop again, never returning to the previous level. The doctors could never confirm why he had the cardiac arrest. They just saw the heart damage and deterioration going forward. There were many medical procedures done on him to extend his life, along with actually getting on and then being removed from the heart transplant list due to his unstable medical condition. I went with him to almost every doctor's appointment, and kept track of his medical records like a woman on a mission. I had Excel files and spreadsheets to track his numbers. I never assumed any one of his doctors knew more about his condition than I did. As his condition worsened, he was given treatment choices. I was there and supported his choices every time, without judgment. Luckily, I had unwavering support from both my nurse-trained sisters, and my parents, otherwise I would not have been able to give my husband that kind of help.

In retrospect, I spent many of those first few months after his passing second guessing the decisions we made and wondering if things would have turned out for the better if we had chosen option B instead of option A. But we can't go back in time, we can only move forward. After some timeI finally realized why I dwelled on it for so long—I survived and he didn't, end of story.

One pleasant memory from his last year on Earth was taking him to a doctor's visit in Vancouver in my recently acquired convertible. It was a warm and sunny September as I threaded us through traffic. I remember looking over at him in the passenger seat, and his head was back, his eyes were closed, and he was enjoying the sun on his face. I still hold that picture of him in the passenger seat and the joy he felt on that day. Unfortunately, things started to unravel quite quickly after that.

In that last year of his struggles with his heart disease, I think... no, I knew that he probably wouldn't make it. I chose to deny it outwardly, but inwardly was a different story. But I still refused to give up hope, if not for me, then for the sake of the kids. He was no longer the man I met, fell in love with, had children with, and would grow old with. It was like looking at an older version of him, aged, withering, withdrawn. My children, now sixteen and thirteen, could see this as well, and unknowingly treated him more like their grandfather living in our home, than their own father. Our mourning of "the loss of him" started long before his actual passing.

I remember his last Christmas in our home. We had to move heaven and earth to get him out of the hospital and home in time for Christmas. But it was not as we had hoped. At first he was happy, but then he became distant and distracted. Like he had run out of whatever energy he had saved up for the holiday. Not long after that, he was in and out of the hospital regularly.

My husband never spoke with me about his possible death, not ever. And I could not bring myself to move from the position of hopeful, to practical. Hence, we never spoke about his estate, his funeral arrangements, anything. I only learned about some of those things, after his death, from the social worker. One of the most uncomfortable decisions that the doctor posed to me, near the end of his life, was the unapproved DNR. Now for those of you not in the know, that is Do Not Resuscitate. It is not a decision to be taken lightly and can have all sorts of emotional baggage attached to it. He was not prepared to authorize it himself. I was afraid to ask him what he wanted. I did not want to be the one that "pulled the plug." Luckily for me, the doctors made the decision themselves.

My husband had been in hospital for a couple of months straight, trying to get his condition stabilized. The hospital called and said that it might be best if myself and the kids came over to visit him. He was not doing well and could use some cheering up. I immediately pulled the kids out of school, we hopped on a float plane and headed over to Vancouver. The doctor's showed me his medical records and said he was likely not going to survive much longer. His immune system had collapsed, he had contracted the dreaded superbug, and antibiotics were no longer working for him. This was a blow, to say the least.

Luckily, I had brought with me twenty-seven years worth of annual Christmas letters that I had been sending out to friends and family. We sat in his hospital room and I had the boys read them out to him. We laughed, we cried, we remembered. At one point, my husband had my oldest son fix the clock in his room, which was hanging crooked. Things seemed almost normal. Almost. During our visit, my husband got tired and fell asleep. We knew we had worn him out with all the memories, and the boys and I left for the hotel that I had booked for us. I was mentally prepared to do the same thing every day, until the end.

But to my complete surprise and shock, I received the call that night that he had passed in his sleep. One part of me was very sad and devastated, but another part was very grateful. I knew deep down, keeping him alive was a form of torture, especially when I saw the number of machines needed to keep him alive. My only regret from that night was not going to the hospital to say my goodbye to him. That night, I chose to stay with my kids; I knew they needed me more than he did.

It wasn't until the next day that I fully realized my state. I'd had a third of my identity ripped out of me. I was now a widow—no longer a wife. I still was Elaine and a mom, but there was a hole where the wife part had lived. What would fill that? Who was I without him? I thought I had prepared myself for this eventuality, but in fact, I was totally and completely unprepared. "The Elaine" I had, was the young, inexperienced, vulnerable one. I came to the realization that I would have to update, refine, or expand the "Elaine" part of me, to fill the void.

I could not do this alone. I needed help. During the process of filling myself with expanded "Elaine," my friends and even my own children encouraged me to get out there and even start dating! The thought of this scared the hell out of me, to say the least. My children decided to get their two cents in and came up with a dating criteria list for me—the attributes of the man I could date with their approval. I decided to add my two cents, and we were off to the races, so to speak.

My short lived time spent on the dating app, Plenty of Fish, was memorable, and may be featured in a future chapter. Needless to say it was a bust, but did help me figure out who the "new me" was. What I liked, what I didn't like. I was starting to find my new voice, my new image.

During this process of repair and transformation, I was reacquainted with a friend of my late husband's. It had been suggested to me by my grief counselor, to create my own grief support group. To collect widows and widowers, for various purposes. I was afraid to collect male widowers who had remarried, since their spouses might think I was "shopping for a new husband." Widows seemed to be in short supply in my network so when a widower came across my radar that hadn't remarried, he, my late husband's friend, was the answer to my prayers. I picked his brain so much I am surprised I didn't empty it. I shared so much with him. He was so easy to bounce things off of. This was all great in the beginning, but then we started dating. He already knew a lot of my quirks and idiosyncrasies that you don't normally share with a person you have just started dating. I felt exposed. I have no idea why we work, since he failed my "dating criteria-dos and don'ts list" but that is okay, I failed all the items on his list too. I started out looking for someone to just talk and dance with (part of my Plenty of Fish profile) and ended up with much, much more—a second chance at true love. We don't try to fill each other's lost loved one's shoes, but to walk beside each other on our own. I'm grateful that destiny put him in my path. He is someone to love for the next chapters in my life.

I can still remember those first couple of months after my husband's death, dreading going into a bank or a government office and explaining that I was there to remove my late husband's name off some account or another. I would see the look of sadness in their eyes when they realized they were dealing with a widow, and I hated that label. Even today, I don't like it. It reminds me of a time when I thought I would be "broken" forever, but luckily that was not true.

A couple of years after my husband's passing, and when I officially retired from my accounting job, I made a list of what I was going to do to fill those work hours with new things. In the beginning, I was still in survival mode, I could not imagine anything too big. Any idea that my life could be bigger than what it was at the moment was beyond my capability. But as each year came and went, I would look at last year's list, and revise it. I have done this now continuously for eleven years. Many things have been accomplished. Some new have been added, but also some have been deleted. Through it all I have learned to face my fears, and make mistakes. *How else can we learn?* But the one thing that I know is that I could never have predicted fourteen years ago that I would be where I am today.

Before my husband's passing, a girlfriend convinced me to go to a belly dance class with her. She made me promise to try it for a month. Now I had tried ballet, jazz, and tap in the past and wasn't good at any of them, so my opinion going in was that I was going to suck at yet another dance genre. But to my surprise, this one stuck. Not only did it stick, but it provided a wonderful way to express any pent up stress that was in my body. I could shimmy until I collapsed and exorcized the worry-demons that seemed to be constantly in my head. This weekly ritual worked so well I created a similar space in an outbuilding on our property. When things seemed to get totally overwhelming, I would go out there and work it off by belly dancing. To this day, I can get so totally caught up while dancing alone that the stresses of the world disappear, at least until the end of the belly dance song.

From that exposure to belly dancing, was born a passion and a small business. Two years after my husband's passing, and at the ripe old age of fifty-one, I started a contemporary belly dance teaching and performing business called, Belly Laughs Navel Academy. It has been an amazing adventure that never in my wildest dreams could I have foreseen. It has taken me outside of my comfort zone so many times I don't even remember what my old comfort zone looked like.

I will always remember the years my husband and I and our two lovely boys spent together, but I did eventually realize that life must go on, if not for the sake of myself, but my boys. I have never avoided or shied away from talking about him with them. We even have this crazy ritual that we try to do around the date of his last day on this Earth. It comes from a funny incident that happened during our vacation in Disneyland. My husband could only drink his coffee with flavored Coffeemate. He used to take a couple of them with him from the hotel to the theme park so he could drink coffee during the day. We went on the Raiders of the Lost Ark ride, and it was so bumpy, the creamers broke open in his front shorts pocket. Well you can imagine the boy's reaction to that. So each year, I get hold of coffee creamers and we smash them open in remembrance of that vacation and the wonderful time we had with him. The boys remind me of their dad quite regularly. Which startles and amazes me, at the same time.

But from my husband's first heart attack to his deteriorating health over the years to his eventual passing, was all a wake up call. Life is fragile; there is no guarantee how much time we have. The only thing we have control over is how we choose to spend it. Mine involved a change in trajectory, or should I say path. Trajectory insinuates that you are out of control, which I am not. Though some years I look back and say, "Wow that was a wild ride," but with a smile on my face not a look of horror—thankfully. I am either a student or a teacher, depending on the moment.,and this works for me; always moving forward.

If any of you reading this are currently going through a period of loss and grief, whether it is because of the death of a loved one or a relationship, if you feel like a piece of you is missing, and you have lost part of your identity—just know that, you have it in you, the ability to remake, to remold, to refill yourself. You are brave enough, you are strong enough to get past whatever life throws at you. It is not about just surviving the ordeal, but thriving.

I am not asking you to forget your past, but to add to it, boldly and with purpose. Make your own list, and start checking things off. As far as what to put on there, the sky's the limit. Start now. We never know how long we have left on this big crazy planet. So let's make the most of every breath we take, from this moment on. I know I will.

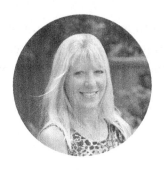

ELAINE DE ROOY

Elaine De Rooy is the proud owner of a contemporary belly dance teaching and performance business in *the highest median age city in all of Canada*, Qualicum Beach, B.C.

Before embarking on this amazing and unexpected path, she witnessed first hand the sudden illness, the five year life and death struggle, and eventual passing of her spouse of twenty seven years. She was left with two active teens and a life she didn't know how to live. Becoming a widow at the age of forty-nine, was not something she was prepared for, in the slightest. She felt like a ship without a rudder, being tossed in a strong and relentless sea. What she really wished for was either a navigator, or someone to throw her a life preserver. Incredibly, she got both her wishes. It came in the form of a fellow widower, and a new unexpected direction in her life, belly dancing. You can connect with Elaine directly at: www.bellylaughsnavelacademy.ca.

Photo credit: Gordon Lafleur Photography

Have the audacity to be curious and believe in yourself.

Sensitivity Advisory: This chapter references personal experiences of substance abuse and sexual violation.

CHAPTER TWELVE

Believe in Your Wildest Dreams

Written by Emma Lewis

We only get one shot at this life. No matter what is happening, no matter where we come from, the circumstances life hands us or challenges we move through —there is always a silver lining: Life is happening for us, not to us.

As I sit on the plane in early September 2024 and write this book chapter on my way home from an epic solo adventure to Scottsdale, AZ, I have equal moments of being so grateful that I ended up here and pinching myself that this is even real. *Am I living a dream?* The answer is yes, I am living a dream; it's the dream I created for myself. But it wasn't always this way, I used to long for this version of my life. Fully funded solo travel with the luxury of time freedom and the joy of my own company, grounded in who I am, emotionally connected with my family, self-aware enough to be able to make new connections with others, able to speak up and believe that my voice and my dreams matter and were possible, it all used to be a daydream of "one day". I was never immune to hard work, but for some reason it always felt like a grind when I worked shift work, struggling to always just get by, and couldn't wait for a day off. I would do it because I knew deep down that no one was coming to save me except myself and I was working towards something bigger than my current circumstances. I used to long for the days where I had the ability to control my own schedule, work anywhere I wanted, and have fun making an impact in my community. Now this is becoming my reality, the evidence which reinforces my belief that anything is possible.

This morning started by waking up in an ultra-comfortable, bougie king-size bed at the Fairmont, Princess Scottsdale resort—a dream. Waking up at six a.m, throwing on my bathing suit, making my morning tea, and wandering down the meandering cement path to the pool. Getting into the pool with what felt like warm bathwater, still felt cooler than the 35 degree celsius ambient air—refreshing. I relaxed into a floating hammock and watched the sunrise over the mountains in the distance. The warm sun beaming off my face and the light glistening off the pool like a shimmering crystal.

There was a six-foot-wide water feature in the middle of this pool with a fire pit on the top. It was enormous and gorgeous. And with the sound of the water trickling into the pool like a waterfall—it was blissful. This was the perfect way to end an amazing trip. I closed my eyes and went into a deep meditation of gratitude that I ended up here—*how is this even real?*

I love my parents dearly and have utmost respect for their own journey in this life, but like me, they too are on their own evolution of growth. They both have grown immensely and are in a much different place now than when our journey started together. When they were raising me, they did the best they could with the skills, knowledge, awareness, and emotional IQ they had access to. They operated in life how they were brought up and exhibited similar relational behaviors that were demonstrated to them. This is understandable, but not ideal, as they both came from dysfunctional families. I bring this up not to bring shame or blame to them, simply to shed light on the environment I was born into.

I know without a doubt that my parents love me, and I am the center of their world. From the outside looking in, we were an average middle class family and had all our basic needs met. There were many moments of happiness and it looked like we were "put together." In reality, this was often a facade to keep the peace. The truth is, I was born into a home that was chaotic, argumentative, toxic, and the words "boundaries" or "respect" were not part of the vocabulary. Both my parents were hard working entrepreneurs and worked their butts off to put food on the table. My dad, a contractor who also made custom wood signs on the side and sold them at a market on the weekend, has struggled with alcohol since before I was born. My mom, a former bank teller and store owner, went back to school to start her own web design and record scanning business when I was five years old. As a recovering people-pleaser, she kept her emotional walls up and was in a constant state of survival around my dad, and by extension me too. My parents both displayed unconscious behaviors of codependency and I often felt a lack of emotional connection with them, which is uneasy for any child to be in. I was very shy and hyper-sensitive as a child, constantly trying to figure out where I fit in or what to do in each moment. Due to the unsettled nature of our home, I unconsciously lived in consistent hypervigilance which cranked my radio dial of awareness for my own safety to the max. Like an antenna on an insect, I was always trying to predict my parents' next moves. It was hard to tell if my dad would explode in anger or be more fun-loving when influenced by alcohol, and it was often difficult to read my mom's body language when she was constantly tense and ready to argue with him. In some ways, this made me grow up too fast, too soon. As our home was "other focused" instead of "child focused", I unconsciously took on emotional caretaking of both parents for the sake of my own belonging, which informed my inner world that my needs didn't matter, or that I even had any.

I wasn't conscious of this at the time, but I spent most of my early years confronted by big emotions figuring out how to survive in this environment, thinking that being in this state was normal. I thought that all my friends experienced walking on eggshells in their homes, too. I thought all parents constantly fought about money, slammed doors, gaslighted each other, and kept grudges for weeks. It felt like our home was in a constant state of turmoil with a sense that an argument could happen any moment always lingered under the surface. *Why did everything have to be so hard at home?* Thanks to my survival skill of hypervigilance, I learned to be an angel child of behavior. Hypervigilance taught me how to stay safe. We now know through Gabor Mate's work that a child has two needs: authenticity and belonging. When their safety—emotional, physical, spiritual or otherwise, is threatened, they will unconsciously choose belonging over authenticity everytime because their survival in the family unit depends on it. Looking back, hypervigilance created the foundational skill of being able to read any situation and comprehend other people's body language or unspoken energy which now contributes to being a great life coach and caregiver.

Even though I behaved well, the misalignment in the home environment came out at school. I started to feel dumb because I struggled with basic math and reading skills to the point where my mom had to get me a tutor. I still remember how to spell "because" properly thanks to the spelling song, "big elephants can always use some exercise," the tutor taught me pops into my head every time I write the word. My report cards were mediocre at best which didn't help my self esteem. My mom had high hopes of me going to trade school; however, university seemed like a distant dream. Becoming a trapeze artist in Cirque du Soleil seemed more and more exciting because I wouldn't have to do this "school stuff."

It wasn't until I started going to friends' houses and seeing how their families interacted that I started to question my own. *Why did I feel more calm outside the home instead of inside?* This is when I started to figure out something wasn't right, my environment wasn't normal. I could sense this but I couldn't put words to it as a young child.

This is not something that as a young child you know how to talk to your parents about, so instead you turn to what you have to soothe the incongruent feelings you're trying to make sense of. For me that was playing Barbies in my room alone dreaming about how life could be different. It also brought me great joy to give my dolls a personality through my imagination and play house in the treefort my dad built me. Upon self reflection, I realize that I started to believe very young that a different reality was possible based on how different I felt in other environments.

As I got older, I turned to sports, music, and gymnastics to calm my inner world. These activities gave me a sense of community, connection, and were an outlet for me to release the emotions locked inside from the uncertainty that was my home life. Sports allowed me to get my feelings and frustration out and to channel my anger and resentment to something more productive. Being part of a team was great for my nervous system to co-regulate with other regulated peers, and gave me and my teammates something to work toward and be proud of—something to believe in. My coaches were consistent and felt like a safe place for me to land. They gave me guidance on the court or the field; but their words impacted me in real life equally, if not more than the playing field. Sports helped me to curate and test the belief I had in myself to do something hard and win. Slowly, I transferred these skills off the court and into my real life.

When I was eleven, the fighting between my parents got so bad that it was to the point of being unsafe. After many therapy sessions, my parents split up and my mom and I moved into a townhouse in the city, leaving my dad in the country. It was hard and emotional and messy, but that was the turning point in all of our lives. Like a fresh canvas, we got to reinvent ourselves and leave behind the tumultuous past, not an easy task but it gave us hope for a better life. My mom knew that she needed help, that there had to be a different way of raising a family. She started seeking help from the community, which led her down a path toward self-help books and personal growth, eventually going to weekend retreats with the top leaders in this space. Her courage and audacity to find a different way catapulted us down a completely different path in life. My mom didn't have childcare at the time, so she brought me with her to many of the events and workshops she attended. Reflecting back, this was a blessing in disguise as my young sponge of a brain got to soak in all the wisdom that people don't usually learn until far later in life, or sometimes at all. Being in these rooms fascinated me and gave me a sense of belonging. I finally started to understand how to have healthier relationships and I gained the belief that my life could be different if I started thinking and acting a different way.

After my parents split, I switched schools in grade 7, which changed the entire trajectory of my future. It is amazing what happens to a child when they are given a different environment and a complete Rolodex of resources to best suit their learning needs. My home life was mostly calm and balanced for the first time in my life. I could focus on my higher learning without my survival brain hijacking my mind all the time and I started to thrive. The positive feedback in my grades kept me wanting to work harder to see what else I was capable of –I started to really believe in myself. By grade 8, the new school approached my mom to advise her that they thought I should be in the advanced placement (AP) class. I am pretty sure that my mom almost fell over hearing this! I flourished in this program and by grade 9 I was accepted into the International Baccalaureate (IB) program that my school had attained accreditation for. The IB program is similar to university but in high school. It is a level higher than AP classes, where in grade 12 you write international exams in hopes of obtaining first year university credits. I wanted to do IB because I knew through the personal development work that I had done that pushing myself in education was the way to a successful life and more opportunities. I knew it would be hard as I am the kid who has to study their butt off to get good marks, but I wasn't afraid of hard work; I believed that I could do it. Even though I didn't end up getting any university credits in the end, IB helped me develop the work ethic required for university and taught me how to think as a sovereign being, how to take initiative on projects, and how to think outside the norm to find solutions. I started to really become someone and believe in who I was. This was in complete opposition to the small, lackadaisical thinking and skimming through school with minimal effort to just to pass the class as a younger child.

At sixteen my mom took me to see Tony Robbins in Toronto at Unleash the Power Within. *And yes I did the fire walk!* There were thousands of people there, all hyped about how amazing this life can be if you choose to create it that way. I had never seen anything like it. Tony said into the mic, "Who here is willing to do whatever it takes and master their mind so they can have or do whatever they desire in life...say I." I got full body chills as an electric rumble went through the stadium as thousands of people yelled "I." At one point, Tony asked anyone in the audience below the age of thirty to stand up. A few hundred people stood up. Then he asked those who were standing to sit down if they were over twenty. There were only a handful of people left standing and I was one of them. I had a split second standing there where I knew this was a catalyst moment, I was on a different path now and there was no turning back. I knew that life could be great, meaningful, peaceful and better than I could imagine. I had to get into rooms with the right people and start thinking differently. I had to believe that it was possible to live the life of my wildest dreams. I had to have the audacity to dream bigger, and then take aligned action towards it. I turned to my mom and said, "I want to be on stage like Tony Robbins one day"!

From that day on, my mom taught me through Wayne Dyers' Book, "You will see it when you believe it," that if I believed in myself, truly feeling it to the core with every cell in my body, I could do anything I set my mind to. It wouldn't matter who doubted me, what obstacles I came across, nothing would be able to stop an audacious woman who believed in herself when no one else did. You start becoming the future version of yourself. If I survived the childhood I had and was okay, I could conquer anything else I put my mind to. My mom and I started learning about everything we could from neuroscience to manifesting, human behavior to trauma. This challenged our limiting beliefs and survival behaviors. I started understanding why I was the way I was. I realized that so much good had come out of the environment that I had deemed bad. I wouldn't be the woman I am today without every single thing that happened to me. I became fascinated with the magnificence of the human body, behavior and the mind/body connection. My career options expanded to wanting to be some kind of therapist instead of a trapeze artist! If I was able to believe in and elicit change in my own life and see results, I wanted to help other people believe they could elicit change too.

With this new fascination with the human body, I had the courage to look for a university. In grade 10 my mom and I flew to Calgary, AB, rented a car, and drove to Vancouver, BC. Along the way we visited all the universities in sight. While at University of British Columbia Okanagan (UBCO) in Kelowna I had an overwhelming feeling of peace and calm. An inner knowing from my intuition that I would attend this school one day. I was in grade 10 and hadn't even graduated high school, but I knew in my soul that I'd be there one day. My mom took a picture of me sitting by the red brick, double tiered water fountain with the UBCO logo in the background. I printed the photo out and stuck it on my wall as a constant reminder to believe in my dreams. I would sit in my room after school and practice what Tony Robbins, Jack Canfield, and Wayne Dyer had been teaching me all along; I wanted to see if it worked. I would feel into what it would be like to be a UBCO graduate, one of the most prestigious schools in Canada at the time. I would imagine flying across the country, moving into my new apartment, smelling the freshly printed paper of my textbooks as I cracked open the cover for the first time, and what it would feel like sitting in a massive lecture theater for my morning biology class. Years before, I was just barely skimming through school dreaming about recess, and now this new possibility of university was becoming more real by the day.

In grade 12 I applied to multiple universities, even though I knew I was going to UBC Okanagan. I still remember the day the UBCO acceptance letter came flying through the mail slot in a massive white envelope with lime green and navy blue writing on it. "Little envelopes are bad news, big envelopes are good news" moved through my mind like a teleprompter as I recalled a teacher telling me that once. Before opening it, I knew that this was my golden ticket. *Nervecited*, equally nervous and excited, I ripped the envelope open and devoured the precious words typed on the cream-colored paper. "Congratulations Emma, you have been accepted into the Human Kinetics Program at UBC Okanagan!" I skipped and sang and danced with joy all around the house. I knew it! I knew that I could do it. Bye, Mom!

Moving from Ontario to British Columbia was one of the best things that I ever did for myself. I moved to B.C. for school, yes, but I also chose to move here to start my life as an adult on my own terms, without the added drama of my family life. Some may call this running away; I call this a fresh start. Moving to B.C. pushed me in ways that I didn't know I needed to be pushed. It forced me and my family to communicate better, because we had to, to stand on my own two feet—to take responsibility and figure out life.

Moving across the country allowed me to decide what I wanted for my life on my own terms. I had a new sense of freedom to be my own person. It was proof to myself that, no matter what happened previously, I could do or have anything that I wanted in life if I really put my mind to it and took action. I moved across the country on my own to attend university, worked full-time to pay for my school, and created a new life and friends here. I was as high on life as I had ever been. I was finally finding my way and figuring out who I wanted to be.

The day I got accepted to university, I remember thinking how grateful I was that I was able to find a new path from the one that was my early childhood. Everyone's life is a complete reflection of the thoughts they think and subsequently actions they take, not their circumstances. Had my life continued on the same path things could have been so much worse for me and my life would have turned out completely differently. Instead, I listened to my intuition and took the path less traveled as an adolescent, met my trauma with curiosity, and asked it what it was here to teach me. I knew from a very young age, with every fiber in my being, that there had to be more to life than just cyclical patterns of abuse and alcoholism, ear-piercing fighting, and dysfunctional relationships. I knew from experiencing the home lives of my friends and the imaginative stories I played out with my dolls that things could be different for me—that there was more. I was determined to figure out what the other people were doing differently than my family.

Then, on the night of my nineteenth birthday, I was sexually abused by someone I thought was a friend. After a typical dorm party in my room, electrifying dance music, and multiple rounds of beer pong, I went to bed so drunk that I could barely function. This behavior was unlike me, but part of the first year university experience. A friend from down the hall, who knew I was wasted, snuck into my room in the middle of the night to "check on me." Instead, he actually had other intentions and proceeded to take advantage of the situation and sexually abuse me. I have vivid memories of yelling at him to stop, but I was so drunk that I blacked out. The next morning, I woke up to the smell of beer and his clothes all over my floor –I was mortified. It all came rushing back to me. In that moment I was flooded with emotions and images of the night before, but I had an unwavering knowing deep in my soul that I was never going to allow this moment to define me or take me off my path to greatness. The severity of the situation definitely had the power to do that, but I would never let it. I trusted that the universe had something bigger instore for me and that this situation was here to teach me something. I immediately checked myself into the school clinic. I got fully tested and booked multiple therapy sessions to work through my pain, betrayal, and devastation.

I never wish this repulsive behavior on anyone. However, this situation did force me to take a really hard look in the mirror. I had to take responsibility for my part in the situation and own where I was acting out of integrity. A hard pill to swallow, but a necessary one. I am not implying that this was my fault and I don't condone this disgusting behavior, but there had to be accountability taken on my part for the unconscious patterns and childhood trauma running on autopilot in the background of my life which caused me to even be in that situation in the first place.

This helped start unraveling the enmeshment and codependency with friends and family I learned as a child, and created paradigm shifts that would set me free for the rest of my life. I am grateful now because even though this is part of my experience, and I have compassion for that part of myself, the sexual abuse does not own me; I own it. Through alternative healing methods, I was able to learn how to transform the negative energy of the experience into liberation and have complete control of how I let it impact my life or not. The freedom of that is more empowering than anything. Finding the silver lining through this made me feel like I could do anything. Your circumstances don't define you, you do.

I found yoga through this experience and it became a huge part of my self-care routine. I fell in love with yoga —so much so that I fulfilled a dream and took my first big solo adventure and traveled to Bali after I graduated university to complete my two hundred hour Yoga Teacher Training (YTT200). One morning my yoga teacher said, "You sit in your stuff, you do the hard asanas (poses), you explore your edges of emotion on the mat so that you get comfortable with the uncomfortable. The more you do this, the easier it will be to apply the same principles off the yoga mat and embody them into your real life." It dawned on me why I loved this practice so much; it made everything in my life so much easier because I was able to sit in the present moment of whatever was in front of me. Doing the hard work in the present made me trust that my future self could fulfill any situation with grace and ease.

Learning how to neutralize the negative energy I experienced in my life and transform it into productive energy or growth, is a superpower. The

Dali Lama once said, "Trees can withstand the most intense storms, but they can't grow roots on the day of the storm. It takes years of daily growth and practice to develop those roots."

The diverse amount of experiences and struggles that I have been through have given me a unique skillset to help others. This ultimately led me to fulfilling my dream of becoming a life coach through Health Coach Institute and furthered my education to become a tools certified life coach through The Life Coach School. During my life coach training, my coach, Brooke Castillo, said something that has really impacted the way I live now. She said, "Why not live your life every day trying to blow your own mind so that you can show your future children what's possible?" I think about this daily, especially when life gets hard, to keep me anchored to my dreams and taking action.

The morning that I was leaving the Fairmont Princess Hotel in Scottsdale, I ordered my breakfast as room service so I could enjoy this bougie room to the very last minute. When the room service attendant knocked on the door, I answered the door in my wet bathing suit and bare feet. The man looked down and complimented the scribed tattoo on my foot, "Believe," that I got for my twenty-first birthday. I sometimes forget that the tattoo is there as it is just part of me now. In an instant, I had deep gratitude wash over me and a flood of memories rush through my mind from what I came from to where I am now. Tears of joy started to roll down my face as I remembered how far I had come in my life. Right before I went on this solo adventure, I had been sitting in uncertainty, not sure of the next step I wanted to take with my business –I was at an intersection of my life. This trip helped me get more comfortable with the uncomfortable, where I met the edge of my own expansion. Remembering the tattoo and how far I had come in life showered a sense of peace and ease over me. No matter how bad the struggle or circumstance, I was going to be okay because it's exactly where I needed to be. Sitting with the unknown was the first step in the next phase of my evolution.

As I reflect back on my life writing this chapter, I can't help but to feel immense appreciation for the big picture of my life. My little self would be so proud of where I ended up. I didn't know I was going to be a life coach when I was a child; heck, it didn't even exist then! I now see how every little detail of my experience had to happen that way. Each moment fits together and gave me the self-awareness and tools I use now to help women who were just like me. All the circumstances I endured and trials I overcame are perfectly perfect and shaped my who I am today. I wouldn't change my life experiences or who I am for the world. I see the beauty in every moment, even the shitty ones.

I now have the privilege to walk hand-in-hand with women who want to create an extraordinary life for themselves. I am so honored to be able to believe in them and show them what's possible when you have the audacity to be curious and believe in yourself. Remember, your circumstances don't define you, you do!

I want every woman who reads this to know that you have complete control over your life. You are not responsible for what happened to you, but it is your responsibility to take accountability for it, to heal, and to decide who you become from it. Whatever you're going through—no matter how hard or terrible the circumstance, you're going to be more than okay. The universe is always going to be there to catch you. The circumstances might not make sense at the time, but have unwavering trust in yourself that you will find your way and it will make sense in the future. Find rooms of people who you resonate with, especially other women as sisterhood is sacred and potent. Curate a rock-solid belief in yourself. Believe in yourself and your dreams with every fiber of your being and feel into what it would be like to live out your wildest dreams. I promise you that you will blow your mind on what you thought was possible and your one shot at this life will turn out better than you could have ever imagined!

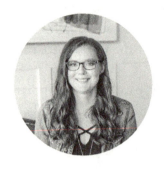

EMMA LEWIS

Born in Ontario, Emma moved to Kelowna, British Columbia for university and has called it home ever since. Emma is a multi-passionate and curious soul who loves to understand the complexities of how things work. You can often find her listening to a podcast or devouring a book on a wide spectrum of health, wellness, or human behavior topics. She loves to connect with others through deep conversation, collaboration, or coaching. In her spare time, Emma lives for traveling and exploring new foods and cultures. She is a bit of an adrenaline junkie and loves new experiences with friends and family. If you're ever in Kelowna, you may run into Emma at a concert, hiking, skiing, or paddle boarding enjoying nature, at the gym during a strength training session, or in the kitchen getting creative with a new food creation or DIY!

If you're interested in reaching out or coaching with Emma, feel free to contact her through her website www.emmalewis.ca.

Never stop believing in your wildest dreams!

It took hearing those words for me to let go of the burden of guilt I had shouldered for more than half a century.

CHAPTER THIRTEEN

The Hummingbird

Written by Heather Goodall

It is not surprising that it was a children's picture book that settled my soul. I am, after all, a teacher who is inspired by beautiful teachings found in books for the young. The Little Hummingbird by Michael Nicoll Yahgulanaas tells a tale of a great fire ravishing the forest. All the other animals were cowering in fear, while Little Hummingbird carried one drop of water at a time from the lake and dropped it on the fire. Bear questioned Little Hummingbird by asking, "What are you doing?" Little Hummingbird replied, "I am doing what I can." It took hearing and sharing those words to my students for me to let go of the burden of guilt I had shouldered for more than half a century.

To really understand the impact of this seemingly simple message there are a few things you need to know about me. As a young child, our dinner conversions did not center around typical parental questions such as, "What did you learn at school today?" "Did you get any tests back or score any goals?" No, my family's question was, "What good deed did you do today?" And not answering was not an option. Yes, we were taught to be kind and to demonstrate that kindness. It really is quite lovely when you think of it. And my mom especially lived by the creed, do unto others. It was taught and expected for myself and my siblings to do good in the world.

I love sharing that antidote because it casts light on the value of putting kindness into the world. But somewhere along the way what got muddled for me was why I was doing good. I came to believe I had to do good, and be good, and give goodness into the world because I owed it to the universe. I grew up with advantages: a loving family, a safe neighborhood, a wonderful group of friends, good health, and opportunities to learn and grow. I could have been in a sitcom from the 1970s.

However, I was not completely sheltered from the ugliness in the world. In 1976, at the age of eleven I attended an international camp in El Salvador, through an organization called Children's International Summer Village (CISV). At the camp there were forty-four children from eleven different countries. It is a non-profit organization that promotes world peace by exposing children to other cultures and fostering international friendships. Seeing the poverty in El Salvador had a profound effect on my understanding of the disparity between the "haves and the have nots." In addition, several months after the camp ended, El Salvador erupted in a civil war, killing or harming many of the people I had connected with.

My privilege was clear. More and more I began to put more pressure on myself. It might sound ludicrous, but not only did I believe that I had to do good, but I needed to do great things with my life because of that privilege. I was influenced by the church and believed wholeheartedly the verse Luke 12:48, "From everyone who has been given much, much will be demanded; and from the one who has been entrusted with much, much more will be asked."

And to be honest, I believed I could do something great. Why not? I was confident, I had drive, I was encouraged by my family to make a difference in the world. And not only that, my destiny was confirmed for me by a Hypnotist Performer at a high school event. I had succumbed to the hypnotist's spell and at the end of the show while still on stage, he whispered to me, "You will do great things!" So there it was, confirmed—I needed to work hard toward changing the world. Now, I wasn't so conceited to think I was great, I just believed I was supposed to do something great. No pressure!

The pressure, albeit perceived pressure, was real. As I navigated my adult years, including a career in education that I loved, raising two girls, running a household, and working at my marriage, I felt like I wasn't doing all that I could to pay my debt for my abundance. Feelings of guilt sometimes sucked the joy out of just living which was accompanied by worry that something bad was going to happen. I questioned how I got so lucky. How is it that I was born into a loving household, in a safe country, with the freedom to live as I wish, with the means to have a house and food? We all know the tragedies and horrors in other countries, we see the homeless in our streets and our hearts break for vulnerable children who are abused and neglected.

So I did more and more to be a giver for my family, community, and school, never saying no. I was driven by my duty, responsibility and yes, guilt. It really was exhausting sometimes, but I had so much abundance in my life that I couldn't waiver and it was unthinkable to ever complain. Thinking nightly, "What good deed did I do today?" Followed by, "Did I do enough?"

On some of those nights, when my mind was in overdrive, I let thoughts of worry creep into my head. *When was it my turn to experience tragedy?* I had a close friend lose a child in a tragic accident. The child who happened to be the same age as my daughter, coincidently with the same name. It was unimaginably devastating for my friend. My heart broke for her. But the feeling I didn't expect was guilt and the thought that if this kind of tragedy could happen to my friend it could happen to me. Again, how did I get so lucky? Guilt is sinister.

And when I was selfish or unkind or greedy, the guilt would feel like a pit in my stomach. Always wanting to do better, to BE better. It was a rabbit hole that I would enter when I was quiet and still for a moment. *Brené Brown,* in her book *Atlas of the Heart,* describes this feeling as "foreboding joy." Being terrified to embrace joy for fear your worst nightmare will come true. In the depths of my being, foreboding joy would invade and strike. It is a terrible predicament to question one's happiness. I was happy, I had, and still have, a wonderful life with more blessings than I can count. But these feelings of being undeserving and unworthy, and sometimes foreboding joy were sabotaging my efforts to be the best version of myself.

Fortunately, there are advantages to getting older. For me it is more time to be still, more wisdom to understand as I reflect, combined with practicing gratitude and giving myself grace. I can think of a few moments that were pivotal in easing the pressure I put on myself. Again, it was a book that spoke to me, *The Five People You Meet in Heaven* by Mitch Albom. After Eddie, the protaganist, dies, he meets people in heaven that he either didn't know well or didn't know at all during his time on Earth. Each of the characters he encounters in the afterlife had been affected by a single choice he had made on Earth. They each shared their story of how they were profoundly affected by Eddie's seemingly benign actions. With every stone we cast, we create a ripple. The outcomes of our actions, whether positive or negative, cannot be controlled. So it really wasn't the grand gestures that mattered most; it was the everyday love and kindness I put out into the world that made a difference.

Now when guilt and self doubt plague my thoughts; "I'm not doing enough, I haven't done enough." I reflect on small moments. Some that seemed so insignificant at the time, but were meaningful and impactful. I recall a conversation I had with a friend who was ill, she was working through trauma and had become anorexic. We met for coffee one day, and I made a comment that she really didn't look that different to me because I just see her, as I had always seen her, as simply my friend. Later she told me how much those words meant to her. At the time, I was not thinking about making her feel better, or trying to "be good or do good." I was only speaking the truth based on my love for her. As naturally as water flows, I was freely loving her with no conscious motive. It was simply a beautiful moment between friends.

I began to recognize other moments that had been shared through a lens of love, not guilt. I can look back on the tragic death of my brother to suicide and know I did what I could when he was alive to show him and tell him I loved him. I felt such sadness. And if I had listened to my inner voice scolding me for not doing enough, I would have crumbled. But knowing I had loved him the best way I could, allowed me to manage my grief and channel his love out into the world.

At my present life stage, I still sometimes grapple with the questions about my motives for giving. *Is it love, guilt, or obligation?* I know when my giving is grounded in love, I am truly happy. I have let go of the pressure to "do better, be better."

There is freedom and peace in knowing that I'm doing what I can. The freedom to set boundaries has been a gift. I have learned to say no. What a revelation! I now know my choices come from a place of love not guilt. I may not be contributing grand acts of greatness, but I am able to give small acts of kindness that will affect others in ways I may never know. I am okay with that now. I have taken the pressure off myself. My mom was right, good deeds are important. And those acts can change the world when they are shrouded in love. The Beatles were correct when they sang, "all you need is love."

My privilege is not defined by what I have, it is defined by what I **get** to give. It is my privilege to have opportunities to shine light into darkness, to extend a hand to those in need, to open my heart in friendship. That is the essence of my journey, like Little Hummingbird. I will continue with love to add a drop of goodness into my world every day.

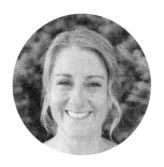

HEATHER GOODALL

As a toddler Heather continually chimed, "Tell me another story," to her Grandmother. Story has been central to her life. She is thrilled to have an opportunity to tell a story of her own. Heather is an educator and one of her greatest joys is teaching children to read. She shares her knowledge and experience with teachers as a literacy leader. Her Educational Consulting Company's, Soul Full Learning: Teaching and Learning with Heart, speaks to Heather's passion and investment in the lives of young people. The two most important young people, who are now adults, are her daughters. They inspire her and fill her soul. Alongside her husband, who champions all her endeavors, Heather continues to do a good deed every day. You can connect with Heather directly at: soulfulllearning@gmail.com.

Photo credit: Ashley Parker

Editor's Note

There is a unique magic and love that every one of Carrie's authors brings to these published collaborations. I often say that Carrie's "people" are the best people, and it is evident throughout this book. It is such an immense joy and privilege to help all these women share their stories. I am deeply touched by reading their words and by getting to work with them over the months to bring this book into the world. I laugh. I weep. I smile and cheer. And when I see the finished chapters, I am filled with so much happiness for these authors that they had the courage to stick with the process. It takes such bravery to be vulnerable in their stories and then allow them to be edited and given feedback. They then have the work of revising their stories to make them even more wonderful for you. It is emotional and oh so beautiful.

Once again, it has been such a pleasure to work alongside all these remarkable authors and collaborate with Carrie to bring their stories to you. Enjoy, darling.

XxM

- Michelle Ireland, Soul Spark Publishing

Author Listing

Carrie Scollon
www.instagram.com/foundher_today

Tisa Sylvester
www.instagram.com/tequissa

Marianne White
www.instagram.com/marianneelizabethdesign

Marnie Law
marnielaw@shaw.ca

Gwen Haas
Gwenseerofthesoul@gmail.com

Erin Gorrie
www.instagram.com/muskokapuppyyoga

Lesa Mueller
www.lesamueller.com

Laura Tolosi
Laura@lauratolosinutrition.com

Miranda Pellett
www.instagram.com/mama24miracles

Paula Campbell
p-campbell@shaw.ca

Elaine De Rooy
www.bellylaughsnavelacademy.ca

Emma Lewis
www.emmalewis.ca

Heather Goodall
soulfulllearning@gmail.com

Acknowledgements

To my incredible sons, you are my greatest source of strength and joy. Through all the challenges, you've been my light and my purpose. This journey hasn't been easy, but every step I've taken has been with you in mind, to give you the best life possible. You've taught me the true meaning of resilience and love, and for that, I am forever grateful. - *Marianne White*

To all the women brave enough to take the next step in witnessing all parts of themselves and especially to Tracy Gawley, my teacher and mentor. Thank you for your guidance and unweaving support. Thank you for bearing witness too and offering me the grace and space to allow the vision of my garden to unfold and blossom. Words can't express my depth of gratitude for all that you've done and continue to do in holding a sacred space for me as I welcome and accept all parts of myself home. - *Gwen Haas*

To my Mom, you were selfless. You never asked for anything. You just gave us what you could, always. It was the biggest honor to walk you home. I love you and will miss you forever. Until we meet again. To my husband, Miles, thank you for being my rock through this journey. Thank you for giving me the opportunity to be where I needed to be and holding me when I need it. I love you. - *Lesa Mueller*

I would like to thank my two boys, Justin and Travis, for giving me a reason to move forward. To my good friend, Sandina, for making me go to those first few belly dance classes. You found me a new passion, belly dance teaching. And to my guy, John, for helping me explore all those new possibilities that I kept coming up with. - *Elaine De Rooy*

I would like to acknowledge and send deepest gratitude to my family and friends. You know who you are. I would also like to send love and light out to those people suffering from leukemia and other cancers, and all of the parents out there in the world who have lost a child, to cancer or otherwise. - *Marnie Law*

To women everywhere who courageously share their stories and engage in brave, sometimes uncomfortable conversations on so many different topics. Your strength and vulnerability shine light on the truth that we are more alike than different. Thank you for your courage and the powerful connections you create by opening your hearts. - *Carrie Scollon*

To all the people who asked the hard questions. - *Tisa Sylvester*

The inspiration for this chapter was me; writing it feels like the final step toward true freedom. I hope it helps to give my boys permission to be gentle with themselves and not let others influence how they feel about who they are. To everyone who has supported me and stood by me on this journey, thank you. - *Erin Gorrie*

To my Mom - Thank you for showing me what beauty looks like on the inside and out. To my daughters - A gift and double blessing in my life. Your beauty shines deep within and I see it every single day in all you do. Keep shining your light, trust and have faith in your body—it is always working for you, and follow what makes your heart strings sing; your path will always be clear. - *Laura Tolosi*

I wish to acknowledge my four miracle babies who have been the shining light needed to get me through the darkest of days. Ameliya, Clara, Jonah, and Lydia—without your unconditional love and faith, I wouldn't have the strength needed to face the highest of mountains and lowest of valleys. You are my whole world... xo. I also need to thank the rest of my family, friends, and our GBS Foundation Family for being the support system we've needed these past eight years. We love you. - *Miranda Pellett*

From the start my mom showed me what it was like to shine a light into this world. I hope, Mom, this story shows that your kindness will continue to ripple to the end of time. - *Heather Goodall*

I would like to thank Carrie Scollon for giving me this opportunity to embark on a journey of writing. Her patience and belief in me, reminded me it is never too late to write and that we need not worry about judgement when our intention is to share our life stories in hopes to inspire others. I will be forever thankful for my parents and our life together, thank you for letting me be me. To my boys who have been my greatest inspiration and for my husband and close friends who know my dreams and push me towards them. - *Paula Campbell*

I dedicate this chapter to my parents who I am full of love and gratitude for. You never stopped believing in me. I love you to the moon and back! I extend my appreciation to the amazing community of friends and family who have been my rock over the past years. Thank you for guiding me up when times were tough and for celebrating my successes. - *Emma Lewis*

About FoundHer

This book has been lovingly brought to you by Carrie Scollon as part of the FoundHer collaborative book series.

At FoundHer, we believe that everyone is inherently enough. Through our podcast and YouTube interviews, summits, retreats, workshops, and book collaborations (just like this one), we empower individuals to discover their passion, purpose, and fulfillment and to embrace their innate worthiness. Our mission is to foster a community where curiosity and imagination lead to clarity and self-acceptance, allowing each person to realize their full potential.

Join us on a journey of self-discovery and empowerment. Embrace your uniqueness and recognize that you are enough. Together, let's unlock the limitless possibilities within ourselves and create lives filled with purpose and fulfillment. Dare to believe that you are more than enough at www. foundher.today.

Writing and Publishing with Soul Spark Publishing

Let's tell your story, darling.

If reading this book ignited a wee spark inside you that has you wondering if you too could write a book and share your story, or if that lingering thought has come back around nudging you that the time to settle in and write your book is now, then we'd love to chat with you about what you have in mind.

Our team works closely with all of our writers to ensure that creating and publishing your book is everything you ever dreamed it could be and that you are so in love with your book that you are proud to share it with the world.

We are by your side from Concept to Publication™ and beyond, so if you dream of becoming a writer and a published author this year, then let's get started at soulsparkpublishing.com or email us directly michelle@soulsparkpublishing.com. We cannot wait to help you tell your story, darling.

P.S. Thinking of putting together your own collaborative book project? We're here for that, too, and love them... obviously. ;)

Contact us at soulsparkpublishing.com or email our Publishing Director, Michelle Ireland, directly at michelle@soulsparkpublishing.com to see how it all works.

Made in the USA
Monee, IL
07 April 2025

14861501R00111